Recent Advances in

SURGERY 39

Recent Advances in
SURGERY 39

Editors

Rachel Hargest MD FRCS
Cardiff China Medical Research Collaborative
Henry Wellcome Building
Health Park Campus
Cardiff University
Cardiff, Wales, UK

Michael Douek MD FRCS
Professor of Surgical Oncology and
Honorary Consultant Surgeon
King's College London and
Guy's and St Thomas' NHS Foundation Trust
London, UK

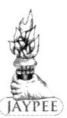

The Health Sciences Publisher
New Delhi | London | Panama

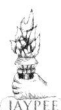 **Jaypee Brothers Medical Publishers (P) Ltd**

Headquarters
Jaypee Brothers Medical Publishers (P) Ltd
4838/24, Ansari Road, Daryaganj
New Delhi 110 002, India
Phone: +91-11-43574357
Fax: +91-11-43574314
E-mail: jaypee@jaypeebrothers.com

Overseas Offices

J P Medical Ltd
83 Victoria Street, London
SW1H 0HW (UK)
Phone: +44 20 3170 8910
Fax: +44 (0)20 3008 6180
E-mail: info@jpmedpub.com

Jaypee-Highlights Medical Publishers Inc
City of Knowledge, Bld. 235, 2nd Floor, Clayton
Panama City, Panama
Phone: +1 507-301-0496
Fax: +1 507-301-0499
E-mail: cservice@jphmedical.com

Jaypee Brothers Medical Publishers (P) Ltd
17/1-B Babar Road, Block-B, Shyamoli
Mohammadpur, Dhaka-1207
Bangladesh
Mobile: +08801912003485
E-mail: jaypeedhaka@gmail.com

Jaypee Brothers Medical Publishers (P) Ltd
Bhotahity, Kathmandu, Nepal
Phone +977-9741283608
E-mail: kathmandu@jaypeebrothers.com

Website: www.jaypeebrothers.com
Website: www.jaypeedigital.com

© 2019, Jaypee Brothers Medical Publishers

The views and opinions expressed in this book are solely those of the original contributor(s)/author(s) and do not necessarily represent those of editor(s) of the book.

All rights reserved. No part of this publication may be reproduced, stored or transmitted in any form or by any means, electronic, mechanical, photocopying, recording or otherwise, without the prior permission in writing of the publishers.

All brand names and product names used in this book are trade names, service marks, trademarks or registered trademarks of their respective owners. The publisher is not associated with any product or vendor mentioned in this book.

Medical knowledge and practice change constantly. This book is designed to provide accurate, authoritative information about the subject matter in question. However, readers are advised to check the most current information available on procedures included and check information from the manufacturer of each product to be administered, to verify the recommended dose, formula, method and duration of administration, adverse effects and contraindications. It is the responsibility of the practitioner to take all appropriate safety precautions. Neither the publisher nor the author(s)/editor(s) assume any liability for any injury and/or damage to persons or property arising from or related to use of material in this book.

This book is sold on the understanding that the publisher is not engaged in providing professional medical services. If such advice or services are required, the services of a competent medical professional should be sought.

Every effort has been made where necessary to contact holders of copyright to obtain permission to reproduce copyright material. If any have been inadvertently overlooked, the publisher will be pleased to make the necessary arrangements at the first opportunity. The **CD/DVD-ROM** (if any) provided in the sealed envelope with this book is complimentary and free of cost. **Not meant for sale.**

Inquiries for bulk sales may be solicited at: jaypee@jaypeebrothers.com

Recent Advances in Surgery 39

First Edition: **2019**
ISBN: 978-93-5270-286-2
Printed at Replika Press Pvt. Ltd.

Contributors

Akshay Anand MS FIAGES
Assistant Professor
Department of General Surgery
King George's Medical University
Lucknow, Uttar Pradesh, India

David Bosanquet MB BCh MRCS MD
Specialist Registrar in Surgery
Aneurin Bevan University Health Board
Department of Surgery
Newport, UK

Charlie Chan MBBS DPhil FRCS
Consultant Breast and General Surgeon
Nuffield Health Cheltenham Hospital
Cheltenham, UK

Michael Douek MD FRCS
Professor of Surgical Oncology and
Honorary Consultant Surgeon
King's College London and
Guy's and St Thomas' NHS Foundation Trust
London, UK

Dorin Dumitru MBBS MS
Locum Consultant Oncoplastic Breast
Surgeon, Hampshire Hospitals NHS
Foundation Trust, Basingstoke
Hampshire, UK
Honorary Specialty Registrar in Oncology
Cambridge University Hospitals NHS
Foundation Trust
Cambridge, UK

Joseph Hardwick PhD FRCS (Plast)
Consultant Plastic Surgeon
University Hospitals of Coventry and
Warwickshire NHS Trust
Warwickshire, UK

Rachel Hargest MD FRCS
Cardiff China Medical Research Collaborative
Henry Wellcome Building
Health Park Campus
Cardiff University
Cardiff, Wales, UK

Richard OS Karoo FRCS (Plast)
Consultant Plastic Surgeon
Welsh Centre for Burns & Plastic Surgery,
Morriston Hospital
Swansea, UK

Sunil Kumar
MS DNB FRCS (Eng) FRCS (Edin) FIAGE
Professor and Head
Department of Surgery
Tata Main Hospital
Jamshedpur, Jharkhand, India

Benjamin JH Lee MBBS
Resident, Department of Surgery
Tan Tock Seng Hospital
Singapore

Joshil V Lodhia MRCS MBBS BSc
Specialist Trainee in
Cardiothoracic Surgery
Health Education Yorkshire and
the Humber, Yorkshire, UK

Rhydian Maggs BSc MSc
Clinical Scientist
Medical Physics Department
Velindre Hospital
Cardiff, UK

Kalnisha Naidoo MB BCh PhD
Guy's and St Thomas'
NHS Foundation Trust and
The Institute of Cancer Research
London, UK

David J O'Regan
MBA MD BM FRCSEd (C-Th) FFSTEd
Consultant Cardiothoracic Surgeon
Leeds Teaching Hospitals NHS Trust
Leeds
Deputy Director, Faculty of Surgical Training
Royal College of Surgeons
Edinburgh, UK

Sotiris Papaspyros FRCSEd (C-Th)
Consultant Thoracic Surgeon
Department of Cardiology and
Cardiothoracic Surgery
Royal Infirmary of Edinburgh
Edinburgh, UK

Sarah E Pinder FRCPath
Professor of Breast Pathology
Cancer Studies
King's College London and Guy's and
St Thomas' NHS Foundation Trust
London, UK

Frank Plani MD FCS (SA) FRACS
Consultant Surgeon
Head of Trauma Unit
Chris Hani Baragwaneth Hospital
Johannesburg, South Africa

Georgiana Samoila MB BCh
Core Surgical Trainee
North West Deanery
Mersey, UK

Paul Shaw
BSc MB ChB MSc DTMH MRCP FRCR PhD
Hon Senior Lecturer
European Cancer Stem Cell
Research Institute
Consultant Oncologist
Velindre Hospital
Cardiff, UK

Vishal G Shelat
MBBS MS DNB MMed FRCSEd FAMS MRCPS FICS
FAIS MNAMS FIMSA MCIHesperis diploma in Organ
Transplantation (ECOT)
Consultant HPB Surgeon
Tan Tock Seng Hospital
Clinical Senior Lecturer
YLL School of Medicine
Singapore

K Sim MBBS
Resident
Department of Surgery
Tan Tock Seng Hospital
Singapore

Anshuman Singh MS
Senior Resident
Department of General Surgery
King George's Medical University
Lucknow, Uttar Pradesh, India

Faris Soliman MRCS
Clinical Research Fellow
Cardiff China Medical Research Collaborative
Cardiff University
Cardiff, UK

Abhinav Arun Sonkar
MS FACS FUICC FRCS (Eng) FRCS (Ire) FRCS (Glas)
Professor and Head
Department of General Surgery
King George's Medical University
Lucknow, Uttar Pradesh, India

Richard M Thomson MRCS MSc
Registrar
Welsh Centre for Burns and Plastic Surgery
Morriston Hospital
Swansea, UK

Arunima Verma MS MRCS(Edin) FIAGES
Consultant Surgeon
Department of Surgery
Tata Main Hospital
Jamshedpur, Jharkhand, India

Christopher Wilcox MB BCh
Clinical Research Fellow
University Hospital Southampton
Southampton, Hampshire, UK

Ian M Williams MD FRCS
Consultant Vascular Surgeon
Cardiff and Vale University Health Board
Cardiff, UK

Acknowledgments

We especially appreciate the constant support and encouragement of Mr Jitendar P Vij (Group Chairman) and Mr Ankit Vij (Group President), Jaypee Brothers Medical Publishers (P) Ltd, New Delhi, India in publishing this book and also their associates particularly Ms Chetna Malhotra Vohra (Associate Director—Content Strategy) and Ms Madhuri Aggarwal (Development Editor) for their expert assistance in the production of this book.

Contents

Section 1: Surgery in General

Chapter 1   Necrotizing fasciitis   3
Richard M Thomson, Richard OS Karoo

Chapter 2   Litigation and how to avoid it?   13
Charlie Chan

Section 2: Training in Surgery

Chapter 3   Acquisition of surgical skills—from novice to master; a fresh perspective   27
Sotiris Papaspyros, Joshil V Lodhia, David J O'Regan

Section 3: Breast Surgery

Chapter 4   Assessment of margins in breast cancer surgery   37
Dorin Dumitru, Michael Douek

Chapter 5   Lobular carcinoma in situ   45
Kalnisha Naidoo, Sarah E Pinder

Section 4: Head and Neck Surgery

Chapter 6   Neck dissection in head and neck cancers   55
Anshuman Singh, Akshay Anand, Abhinav Arun Sonkar

Section 5: Upper Gastrointestinal Surgery

Chapter 7   Penetrating trauma of the upper gastrointestinal tract: Practical notes on surgical management   69
Frank Plani

Section 6: Lower Gastrointestinal Surgery

Chapter 8   Novel radiotherapy techniques for the treatment of anal cancer   85
Paul Shaw, Rhydian Maggs

Chapter 9   Anorectal and perineal manifestations of tuberculosis   94
Arunima Verma, Sunil Kumar

| Chapter 10 | Surgical considerations during pregnancy and delivery in women with Crohn's disease
Faris Soliman, Rachel Hargest | 103 |

Section 7: **Hepatobiliary Surgery**

| Chapter 11 | Pyogenic liver abscess
Benjamin JH Lee, K Sim, Vishal G Shelat | 113 |

Section 8: **Vascular Surgery**

| Chapter 12 | Thoracic outlet syndrome
Georgiana Samoila, Ian M Williams | 125 |

Section 9: **Innovation in Surgery**

| Chapter 13 | The use of three-dimensional printing in surgery
Joseph Hardwicke | 143 |

Section 10: **Clinical Trials**

| Chapter 14 | A review of recent randomized controlled trials in surgery
David Bosanquet, Christopher Wilcox, Rachel Hargest | 157 |

Index   *173*

Section 1

Surgery in General

CHAPTERS

1. Necrotizing Fasciitis
2. Litigation and How to Avoid it?

Chapter 1

Necrotizing fasciitis

Richard M Thomson, Richard OS Karoo

INTRODUCTION AND BACKGROUND

Necrotizing fasciitis is a life threatening, rapidly advancing infection that progresses along fascia and subcutaneous tissues. It is a surgical emergency needing a high index of suspicion, early diagnosis, and aggressive surgical debridement. Delay often increases the risks of mortality.

The term "Necrotizing Fasciitis" can be confusing. Often reports in the media will refer to it as a condition involving "flesh-eating bacteria". It is commonly used as a general term to describe necrotizing soft tissue infections (NSTIs). NSTIs encompass necrotizing forms of cellulitis, fasciitis, and myositis depending of the depth of tissues involved. The term is also used interchangeably with Fournier's gangrene when infection affects the genitourinary tract and Ludwig angina when involving submandibular and sublingual spaces.[1]

HISTORICAL CONTEXT

The first recorded description of necrotizing fasciitis was by Hippocrates in 400 BC.

> "Many were attacked by the erysipelas, it would quickly spread widely in all directions... flesh, sinews and bones fell away in large quantities... fever was sometimes present and sometimes absent... there were many deaths... the course of the disease was the same to whatever part of the body it spread".[2]

In the late 18th century, Leonard Gillespie, a British Naval Surgeon to Lord Nelson who together with two naval physicians, Thomas Trotter and Sir Gilbert Blane, first described the disease in English. It was referred to as hospital gangrene or phagedena.[3,4] Hospital gangrene was the dominant term used and was described by Joseph Jones a United States Confederate Army surgeon in 1871. He reported 2,642 cases occurring in surgical wounds during the American civil war with a mortality rate close to 50%.[5] Fournier's gangrene was first described in 1764 by Baurienne, but later given its eponymous name in 1883 after Jean Alfred Fournier a French dermatologist or venereologist who described five cases of NSTI in the perineal region.[6]

The cause of the disease was identified as a bacterial infection by 1918. The term necrotizing fasciitis was first used by Wilson in 1952, identifying that necrosis of the fascia was a significant feature of the disease.[7]

EPIDEMIOLOGY

Necrotizing fasciitis is a rare condition with an overall incidence of 0.4–1 per 100,000 per year.[8] Public Health England estimates that there are approximately 500 new cases per year in the UK, with a mortality rate of around 25%. There is thought to be a recent increase in incidence, considered to be related to higher levels of reporting and increased bacterial virulence.[9] It affects males and females equally.

RISK FACTORS

Patients will often have pre-disposing risk factors for developing necrotizing fasciitis, most of which are associated with immunosuppression and hospital admission **(Table 1.1)**.[10]

There will frequently be a precipitating cause within the history:
- *Surgery*—especially intraperitoneal infection, incision, and drainage of perianal or perineal abscesses
- *Minor procedures*—intramuscular infections, intravenous cannulation, and joint aspiration
- *Trauma*—contaminated wounds including marine contamination, insect/animal bite, and burns
- *Soft tissue infection*—following Varicella infection in children.[11]

It is important to remember that half of patients developing necrotizing fasciitis will be normal healthy patients with trivial injuries or no evidence of a site of entry.[12]

PATHOPHYSIOLOGY

An understanding of the pathophysiology is important in understanding the clinical presentation of the disease. Necrotizing fasciitis results from the action of one or more bacteria that proliferate in the subcutaneous tissues. Bacteria spread rapidly along superficial and deep fascial tissue planes facilitated by enzymes (hyaluronidase) that degrade the polysaccharides responsible for tissue adhesion. Excretion of exotoxins stimulates the production of cytokines damaging the endothelial lining and causes leaking of fluid into the extravascular space. Reduced intravascular blood flow results in vessel occlusion by microthrombi.[13] Tissues become ischemic resulting in significant pain and causing overlying

Table 1.1: Risk factors for development of necrotizing fasciitis.
- *Immunosuppression*—medication, HIV/AIDS
- *Diabetes*—up to 70% of cases[10]
- *Chronic diseases*—cirrhosis or liver failure, chronic kidney disease, and peripheral vascular disease
- Malignancy
- Intravenous drug misuse
- Obesity
- Age > 60 years

(HIV: Human immunodeficiency virus; AIDS: Acquired immunodeficiency syndrome).

skin necrosis. These hypoxic conditions enable the proliferation of more anaerobic bacteria accelerating the disease process. Anaerobic bacteria produce carbon dioxide, hydrogen, nitrogen, hydrogen sulfide, and methane. These gases accumulate in the tissues, giving rise to the characteristic sign of crepitus and appearance of gas on imaging. The fascia is particularly susceptible to necrosis given it is relatively avascular. Liquification of the fascia is a diagnostic feature. Progression to the deeper fascia of the intermuscular septum and myonecrosis are late signs and indicates poor prognosis. There is microbial invasion of local blood vessels, which together with toxins cause severe sepsis, multisystem organ failure, and death.[14]

MICROBIOLOGY

Necrotizing soft tissue infection including necrotizing fasciitis can be classified into three bacteriological classes, described by Giuliano et al.[15] Some authors have described a fourth category, which is based on fungal infection[16,17] **(Table 1.2)**.[18] Each class tends to affect different patient populations and has typical clinical features. However, there is no difference in clinical course nor mortality between the groups.

Type I (polymicrobial) infections are the most common accounting for 90% of cases. Bacteria act synergistically—the aerobic bacteria causing tissue destruction and hypoxia enabling the anaerobic bacteria to proliferate. Type I infections tend to infect older and immunocompromised patients, such as individuals with diabetes or renal failure. Trauma is often absent, although there is commonly a breakdown in tissue integrity for example following an ulcer or abscess. The *Clostridia* subtypes give rise to gas, hence, the descriptive term *"gas gangrene"* which is now relatively uncommon following improvements in hygiene and sanitation. Historically, it was related to severe trauma, but currently, it is more commonly seen following contaminated abdominal surgery and has been associated with intravenous drug misuse.[19] Toxins (α-toxin and θ-toxin) cause neutrophil dysfunction and platelet adherence causing impaired phagocyte function and hemolysis.[5]

Type II (monomicrobial) infections are less common. Group A β-hemolytic *Streptococci* can evade the body's immune system by expressing M proteins that enable the microbe to adhere to tissue-evading phagocytosis. M proteins also bind to T-cell receptors leading to enhanced inflammatory response with release of interleukins and cytokines resulting in

Table 1.2: Classification of necrotizing soft tissue infections (NSTIs).

	Type I	Type II	Type III	Type IV
Organisms	Polymicrobial: Gram-positive cocci, *Staphylococcus Aureus, Streptococcus Pyogenes Enterococci* Gram-rods, *Escherichia coli, Pseudomonas* Anaerobes bacteroides *Clostridia* species: *Clostridium perfringens Clostridium septicum Clostridium sordellii*	Monomicrobial: Group A β-hemolytic *Streptococci Staphylococcus Pyogenes, Staphylococcus Aureus*, MRSA[18]	Marine organisms: *Vibrio vulnificus*	Fungal: *Zygomycetes Candida*

(MRSA: Methicillin-resistant *Staphylococcus aureus*).

severe sepsis.[20] They typically occur in healthy patients with no significant past medical history. There is frequently a history of trauma, often trivial.

Type III infections are caused by Gram-negative marine organisms typically Vibrio species (*V. vulnificus*). Infection can occur following marine contamination of an open wound.[21]

Type IV infections are caused by fungal infections, including zygomycetes after traumatic wounds or burns and candidal infections in immunocompromised patients. These can be rapidly progressive.[16,17]

CLINICAL FEATURES (FIGURE 1.1)

The diagnosis of necrotizing fasciitis is not always straightforward and requires a high index of suspicion. The presentation will vary depending on the organism responsible, depth of infection, and anatomical location. Patients may present with early features of localized evidence of skin inflammation (pain, erythema, and edema) or present with later systemic symptoms of sepsis (pyrexial, tachycardia, hypotension, tachypnea, and altered mental state). Patients may have predisposing factors in the history and a precipitating cause. Key features are:

- *Pain*—localized to the overlying skin and muscle and beyond the apparent site of infection. Classically, pain is out of proportion to the degree of skin inflammation. It is important to note that pain is reduced in patients with diabetic neuropathy. Skin changes—ill-defined or patchy erythema and edema. Lymphangitis and lymphadenopathy are absent in NSTIs (but are a feature of cellulitis). Skin vesicles or bullae containing serous fluid are specific but not sensitive signs. Crepitus is a late sign and a sinister feature, and presents in less than 20% of cases.[22] Late signs include skin necrosis and a patch of anesthesia over the site of erythema (from infarction of cutaneous nerves) **(Table 1.3)**.[23]
- *Systemic features*—temperature more than 38°C, tachycardia, hypotension, and tachypnea (secondary to acidosis). Diabetic patients can present in diabetic ketoacidosis.

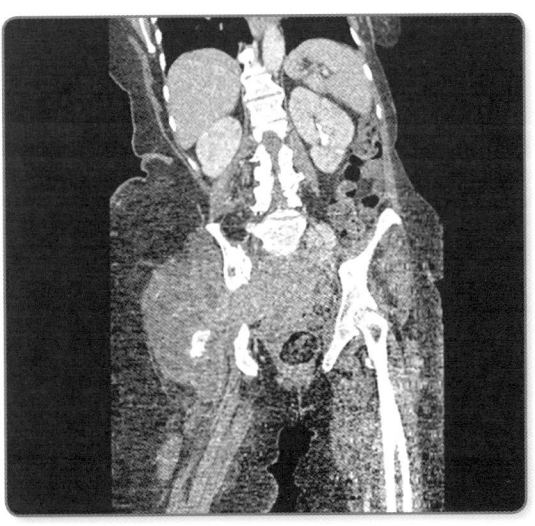

Figure 1.1 Radiograph of thigh showing air in subcutaneous tissue.

Table 1.3: Sites of infection.[23]

Site	Frequency
Lower limbs	28%
Upper limbs	27%
Perineum	21%
Trunk	18%
Head and neck	5%

An important feature of necrotizing fasciitis is the speed of progression, which is usually very rapid. This is in contrast to cellulitis or abscess formation. When the diagnosis is unclear for example during the early stages of the disease, it is prudent to regularly re-review the patient to monitor for signs of disease progression.

INVESTIGATIONS

Necrotizing fasciitis is a clinical diagnosis and a surgical emergency. If it is the suspected underlying diagnosis in a critically ill patient, investigations should not delay surgical intervention. Diagnosis is often made by a combination of visual inspection and digital examination of tissue—the "Finger Sweep Test".[24] An initial incision is carried out in the emergency department or ward under local anesthesia, or in theater under general anesthesia. Examination of the tissues will often reveal:
- Grayish necrotic fascia
- Positive "finger sweep test"—finger can be easily passed between the facial planes
- Presence of a foul smelling purulent discharge often described as "dirty dish water"
- Absence of bleeding of the fascia during tissue dissection.[12]

In cases, where the diagnosis is not clear, laboratory tests and appropriate imaging studies can aid the diagnosis—however, none are diagnostic. The laboratory risk indicator for necrotizing fasciitis (LRINEC) is an effective tool to help distinguish necrotizing fasciitis from other soft tissue infections such as severe cellulitis or abscess.[25,26] Patients are scored on the indicators shown in the Table below in order to predict the risk of necrotizing fasciitis (**Table 1.4**).

The scores from **Table 1.4** are calculated and patients can be classified into three groups as shown in **Table 1.5**.

When the authors used LRINEC more than or equal to 6 as a cut-off for necrotizing fasciitis the positive predictive value is 92% and the negative predictive value is 96%.[25] Although widely used, it is important to note that the tool is not validated or specific to necrotizing fasciitis; other critically ill patients will also score highly. A metabolic acidosis and raised lactate on an arterial blood gas are indicators of critical illness.

IMAGING

Plain film radiography (**Figure 1.2**) can show gas within the soft tissues in the presence of polymicrobial (including Clostridia) infection. This is a nonspecific sign and its absence certainly does not exclude necrotizing fasciitis. Ultrasound can have a role in determining the presence or absence of an abscess and can reveal subcutaneous gas and edema

Table 1.4: Risk predictors in necrotizing fasciitis.

Variable	Value	Points
C-reactive protein (CRP) (mg/dL)	<150	0
	>150	4
WBC (per mm³)	<15	0
	15–25	1
	>25	2
Hemoglobin (g/dL)	>13.5	0
	11–13.5	1
	<11	2
Serum sodium (mmol/L)	>135	0
	<135	2
Serum creatinine (μmol/L)	≤141	0
	>141	2
Serum glucose (mmol/L)	<10	0
	>10	1

Table 1.5: Risk of necrotizing fasciitis.

Group	Score	Risk of necrotizing fasciitis
Low	≤5	<50%
Moderate	6–7	50–75%
High	≥8	75%

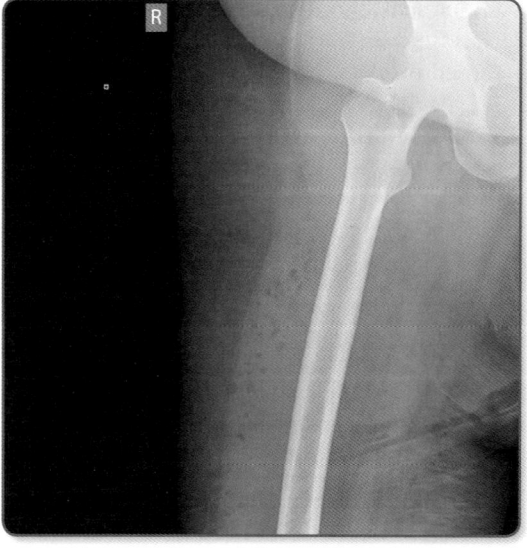

Figure 1.2 Extensive surgical debridement of necrotizing fasciitis of buttocks.

along fascial plains.[27] Magnetic resonance imaging (MRI) scans are highly sensitive, if no fascial thickening is found, necrotizing fasciitis can be excluded. MRI imaging alone can overestimate the extent of deep fascial involvement and should be closely interpreted with clinical findings.[28]

TREATMENT

Necrotizing fasciitis is a surgical emergency and treatment should be initiated immediately. Early operative debridement is the most important determinant of mortality and morbidity. Once necrotizing fasciitis is suspected, empirical intravenous antibiotics together with intravenous fluid resuscitation should be commenced. Early involvement of intensive care specialists is mandatory.

Antimicrobial treatment

The choice of antimicrobials should be discussed urgently with a microbiologist. In our unit, patients are commenced on empirical treatment of intravenous meropenem and clindamycin or metronidazole together with clindamycin and ciprofloxacin in the case of a severe penicillin allergy. In cases with known Group A *Streptococci*, patients are commenced on benzylpenicillin and clindamycin. Meropenem is a broad-spectrum antibiotic covering aerobic and anaerobic Gram-positive and Gram-negative infections. Clindamycin acts to suppress bacterial toxin synthesis with a prolonged effect and has a broad spectrum of action. The process of tissue hypoxia and intravascular thrombosis impedes delivery of antibiotics and necrotic tissues prevent penetration of antibiotics into tissues.

Surgery

Radical surgical debridement is the mainstay of treatment **(Figure 1.3)**. This should be performed by an experienced surgeon. There is good evidence that increased time from presentation to initial debridement and inadequate initial debridement are associated with increased mortality.[12,29,30] Patients should be consented regarding the seriousness of the infection and informed that the risk of mortality is increased without wide surgical excision. Bacteriology swabs and tissue samples should be sent for urgent microscopy and attention of the microbiologist. All infected and necrotic tissues should be excised noting that necrotic fascia often extends beyond the area of affected overlying skin. Inadequate excision will

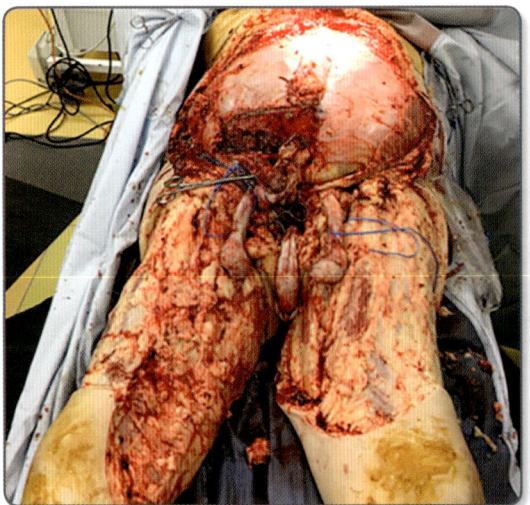

Figure 1.3 Extensive necrotizing fasciitis of buttocks.

allow the disease to progress. Viable tissue can be determined by an incision. If there is any doubt about the viability of the tissue it should be excised. The extent of infected tissue can be large but excision should continue back to healthy bleeding tissue at all margins. Once the surgeon is happy with the extent of the debridement, there should be hemostasis and the wound should be dressed. We use a simple nonadherent paraffin tulle gras dressing (Jelonet, Smith and Nephew), with Betadine-soaked gauze, cotton wool roll or Gamgee®, and crepe bandage. Following surgery the patient should go to an intensive care unit where the team can continue intravenous antibiotics together with supportive treatment and nutritional support. There is always a risk of underestimating disease extent or missing ectopic disease foci, so the patient may be returned to theater within 24–48 hours for a second look, or sooner, if their condition is not improving. At the second look operation any nonviable tissue is excised, the wound is cleaned and redressed. This process continues until the wound is healthy and the patient's condition improves.

Specific anatomical sites

- *Head and neck*—not a common site for necrotizing fasciitis. Reported to follow abscesses in the pharynx. Radical debridement can be challenging given vital structures.[31]
- *Perineum*—subsequent wound care can be challenging owing to fecal contamination. Patients will often require a diverting colostomy although some units manage with regular dressing changes.
- *Upper limb*—need for postoperative splinting.[32]

Reconstructive surgery

Once the patient's condition is stable and the wounds look clean and healthy, attention is turned to reconstruction. In small wounds, it may be possible to achieve delayed primary closure or if appropriate to allow the wound to heal by secondary intention. Topical negative pressure dressings can aid this process. Larger wound management should be in collaboration with a plastic and reconstructive surgeon. Extensive soft tissue loss will often require skin grafting techniques and/or local flaps of tissue for reconstruction and wound closure.

Other adjunctive treatments

There is some limited evidence for the use of intravenous immunoglobulin in necrotizing fasciitis caused by streptococcal infection. It is thought to bind to exotoxins and reduce the systemic inflammatory response.[33]

Hyperbaric oxygen therapy is postulated to increase levels of plasma oxygen above resting tissue oxygen requirements. The patient is enclosed in a treatment chamber and breaths 100% oxygen while at a pressure greater than 1 atmosphere. More oxygen is dissolved in plasma leading to higher tissue oxygen tension in zones of hypoxic tissue, preventing extension of disease, and reducing the need for further debridement. There will also be an associated reduction in tissue edema further improving tissue oxygen tension. Hyperoxia is reported to promote angiogenesis and reduce the growth of anaerobic bacterial species. Although there is physiological rationale, its use remains controversial and there is a lack of robust evidence. Access to hyperbaric facilities is limited often precluding its use in critically ill patients. It is never a substitute for radical surgical debridement.[34]

PROGNOSIS

Without surgery, the mortality of necrotizing fasciitis is extremely high. The prognosis will depend on many factors including underlying medical problems, causative organism, and the speed and extent of surgical debridement. Mortality is reported to be between 6% and 76%.[35]

> **Key points for clinical practice**
>
> - Necrotizing fasciitis is commonly used as a general term to describe a spectrum of NSTIs.
> - Diagnosis of necrotizing fasciitis requires a high index of suspicion—half of patients will normally be healthy with a history of trivial trauma.
> - Necrotizing fasciitis is a clinical diagnosis and a surgical emergency.
> - Radical surgical debridement is the mainstay of treatment.
> - Multidisciplinary working with microbiology and intensive care can improve patient outcome.

REFERENCES

1. Puvanendran R, Huey JCM, Pasupathy S. Necrotizing fasciitis. Can Fam Physician. 2009;55(10):981-7.
2. Descamps V, Aitken J, Lee MG. Hippocrates on necrotising fasciitis. Lancet. 1994;344(8921):556.
3. Loudon I. Necrotising fasciitis, hospital gangrene, and phagedena. Lancet. 1994;344(8934):1416-9.
4. Keevil JJ. Leonard Gillespie (1758-1842); naval surgeon and physician to Lord Nelson. J R Nav Med Serv. 1953;39(4):229-49.
5. Hakkarainen TW, Kopari NM, Pham TN, et al. Necrotizing soft tissue infections: review and current concepts in treatment, systems of care, and outcomes. Curr Probl Surg. 2014;51(8):344.
6. Vaz I. Fournier gangrene. Trop Doct. 2006;36(4):203-4.
7. Wilson B. Necrotizing fasciitis. Am Surg. 1952;18(4):416-31.
8. File TM Jr, Tan JS, DiPersio JR. Group A streptococcal necrotizing fasciitis. Diagnosing and treating the "flesh-eating bacteria syndrome". Cleve Clin J Med. 1998;65(5):241-9.
9. Sarani B, Strong M, Pascual J, et al. Necrotizing fasciitis: current concepts and review of the literature. J Am Coll Surg. 2009;208(2):279-88.
10. Wong CH, Chang HC, Pasupathy S, et al. Necrotizing fasciitis: clinical presentation, microbiology, and determinants of mortality. J Bone Joint Surg Am. 2003;85-A(8):1454-60.
11. Bingol-Kologlu M, Yildiz RV, Alper B, et al. Necrotizing fasciitis in children: diagnostic and therapeutic aspects. J Pediatr Surg. 2007;42(11):1892-7.
12. Childers BJ, Potyondy LD, Nachreiner R, et al. Necrotizing fasciitis: a fourteen-year retrospective study of 163 consecutive patients. Am Surg. 2002;68(2):109-16.
13. Fink A, DeLuca G. Necrotizing fasciitis: pathophysiology and treatment. Dermatol Nurs. 2002;14(5):324.
14. Young MH, Aronoff DM, Engleberg NC. Necrotizing fasciitis: pathogenesis and treatment. Expert Rev Anti Infect Ther. 2005;3(2):279-94.
15. Giuliano A, Lewis F Jr, Hadley K, et al. Bacteriology of necrotizing fasciitis. Am J Surg. 1977;134(1):52-7.
16. Wai PH, Ewing CA, Johnson LB, et al. Candida fasciitis following renal transplantation. Transplantation. 2001;72(3):477-9.
17. Jain D, Kumar Y, Vasishta RK, et al. Zygomycotic necrotizing fasciitis in immunocompetent patients: a series of 18 cases. Mod Pathol. 2006;19(9):1221-6.
18. Miller LG, Perdreau-Remington F, Rieg G, et al. Necrotizing fasciitis caused by community-associated methicillin-resistant Staphylococcus aureus in Los Angeles. N Engl J Med. 2005;352(14):1445-53.
19. Bryant AE, Stevens DL. Clostridial myonecrosis: new insights in pathogenesis and management. Curr Infect Dis Rep. 2010;12(5):383-91.
20. Anaya DA, Dellinger EP. Necrotizing soft-tissue infection: diagnosis and management. Clin Infect Dis. 2007;44(5):705-10.

21. Howard RJ, Pessa ME, Brennaman BH, et al. Necrotizing soft-tissue infections caused by marine vibrios. Surgery. 1985;98(1):126-30.
22. Hsiao CT, Lin LJ, Shiao CJ, et al. Hemorrhagic bullae are not only skin deep. Am J Emerg Med. 2008;26(3): 316-9.
23. Golger A, Ching S, Goldsmith CH, et al. Mortality in patients with necrotizing fasciitis. Plast Reconstr Surg. 2007;119(6):1803-7.
24. Clark R, McGill D. Necrotising Fasciitis: Always use the finger. BMJ. 2005;330:830.
25. Wong CH, Khin LW, Heng KS, et al. The LRINEC (Laboratory Risk Indicator for Necrotizing Fasciitis) score: a tool for distinguishing necrotizing fasciitis from other soft tissue infections. Crit Care Med. 2004;32(7):1535-41.
26. Sandner A, Moritz S, Unverzagt S, et al. Cervical necrotizing fasciitis—the value of the Laboratory Risk Indicator for Necrotizing Fasciitis score as an indicative parameter. J Oral Maxillofac Surg. 2015;73(12): 2319-33.
27. Wronski M, Slodkowski M, Cebulski W, et al. Necrotizing fasciitis: early sonographic diagnosis. J Clin Ultrasound. 2011;39(4):236-9.
28. Schmid MR, Kossmann T, Duewell S. Differentiation of necrotizing fasciitis and cellulitis using MR imaging. Am J Roentol. 1998;170(3):615-20.
29. Voros D, Pissiotis C, Georgantas D, et al. Role of early and extensive surgery in the treatment of severe necrotizing soft tissue infection. Br J Surg. 1993;80(9):1190-1.
30. Bilton BD, Zibari GB, McMillan RW, et al. Aggressive surgical management of necrotizing fasciitis serves to decrease mortality: a retrospective study. Am Surg. 1998;64(5):397-400.
31. Sepúlveda A, Sastre N. Necrotizing fasciitis of the face and neck. Plast Reconstr Surg. 1998;102(3):814-7.
32. Gonzalez MH, Kay T, Weinzweig N, et al. Necrotizing fasciitis of the upper extremity. J Hand Surg. 1996;21(4):689-92.
33. Darenberg J, Ihendyane N, Sjolin J, et al. Intravenous immunoglobulin G therapy in streptococcal toxic shock syndrome: a European randomized, double-blind, placebo-controlled trial. Clin Infect Dis. 2003;37(3): 333-40.
34. Jallali N, Withey S, Butler PE. Hyperbaric oxygen as adjuvant therapy in the management of necrotizing fasciitis. Am Surg. 2005;189(4):462-6.
35. Hasham S, Matteucci P, Stanley P, et al. Necrotising fasciitis. BMJ. 2005;330(7495):830-3.

Chapter 2

Litigation and how to avoid it?

Charlie Chan

INTRODUCTION

All medical practitioners and surgeons are likely to become involved in some form of medical litigation during their careers. The number of complaints increases every year, and doctors face scrutiny from patients, employing hospitals, the Coroner's Court and from our own regulator, the General Medical Council (GMC).

Medical litigation against individual doctor and hospital is increasing, and this chapter will explore the rise in claims, its financial impact, and how this might affect individual surgeons. It will also examine the processes involved in a complaint leading to a lawsuit in the Civil Courts, as well as discussing referral of a doctor to the GMC. Although this chapter is based on English legal practise, similar principles will apply in many jurisdictions worldwide.

MEDICAL INDEMNITY

This is a requirement under section 63 of the *"Duties of a Doctor"*, as published by the GMC. No doctor should practise without indemnity cover, so that patients will not be disadvantaged, if they make a claim about clinical care. This requirement was made statutory in August 2015 following legislation entitled *"The General Medical Council (Licence to Practice and Revalidation) (Amendment) Regulations Order of Council 2015"*.

Doctors practising solely within National Health Service (NHS) hospitals are covered by the NHS Resolution (formerly known as NHS Litigation Authority NHS LA), which was set up 20 years ago. This is funded by contributions under the Clinical Negligence Scheme for Trusts (CNST), where member NHS hospitals pay premiums that are based on the hospital size and its risk profile.

General practitioners (GPs) and doctors practising in the independent/private sector are not covered by NHS Resolution. GPs and private doctors are required to have personal indemnity, which has traditionally been provided by the Medical Defence Organizations (MDOs), such as the Medical Defence Union (MDU), Medical Protection Society (MPS), and the Medical and Dental Defence Union of Scotland (MDDUS). As premiums have increased significantly over the last few years, other companies now offer cheaper medical indemnity products, which differ significantly from the traditional MDO service.

Some NHS care is now provided within the private hospital sector. Some private hospitals make a contribution toward CNST, so that medical indemnity for these NHS cases is covered by NHS Resolution. However, this is not mandatory, and any doctor, considering NHS work within the private sector, should clarify the indemnity situation with the independent hospital and insurer.

In addition to providing indemnity against standard medical claims, the MDOs also provide cover for "Good Samaritan" acts, assistance with employment disputes, and importantly, cover for regulatory proceedings, such as referral to the GMC. Some of the new insurance providers may not provide these extra services offered by the MDOs.

The most important difference between the traditional MDOs and the newer insurance products is the way the schemes are run. The traditional MDOs offer membership or cover provided on an "Occurrence Basis". This means that indemnity is provided for any case treated during that annual subscription year, irrespective of when the claim is made. This is very important, as many medicolegal cases do not occur until several years after the date of treatment and therefore insurance year. This "Occurrence Basis" cover means that members are insured for any claim arising from a patient episode during that year for the rest of the doctor's life, including during retirement.

Some of the newer and cheaper insurance products are based on a "Claims Made" model, which means that the annual premium only provides indemnity against new claims, which have been notified during the year of that insurance. This means that cover is only provided until the end of the annual premium. The premium in these new schemes provides a fixed amount of cover, usually £10 million, as opposed to the discretionary amount of cover provided by the MDOs. While a "Claims Made" premium is cheaper, it does mean that doctors will need to purchase separate run-off cover when they retire, so that they continue to be indemnified against any subsequent claim. Failure to do so can mean that the doctor will have to fund the legal costs and entire claim out of the doctor's individual pocket, which can be ruinous.

RISE IN MEDICAL LITIGATION

The number of new medicolegal claims continues to rise inexorably. This does not necessarily mean that doctors are less competent than before. There are other significant reasons, such as greater public awareness about litigation, more willingness for patients to consider suing, and increased availability and access to legal help through advertising, conditional fee arrangements, and funding through some household insurance policies.

New NHS Resolution claims have doubled over an 8-year period **(Figure 2.1)** and the number of MPS claims has increased by nearly 40% over 6 years.

Over the same time period, the total annual cost of clinical claims for NHS Resolution has risen from £633.4 million in 2007/08 to £1488.5 million in 2015/16 **(Figure 2.2)**. Costs have gone up similarly for the traditional MDOs as well over this time period.

COMMON REASONS FOR MEDICAL LITIGATION

- Delayed diagnosis
- Inadequate consent—an increasing problem
- Communication issues
- Treatment problems, e.g. surgical errors
- Inappropriate delegation leading to mistakes in patient care—be aware of your own and your junior colleague's limitations
- Medication errors.

Common reasons for medical litigation   15

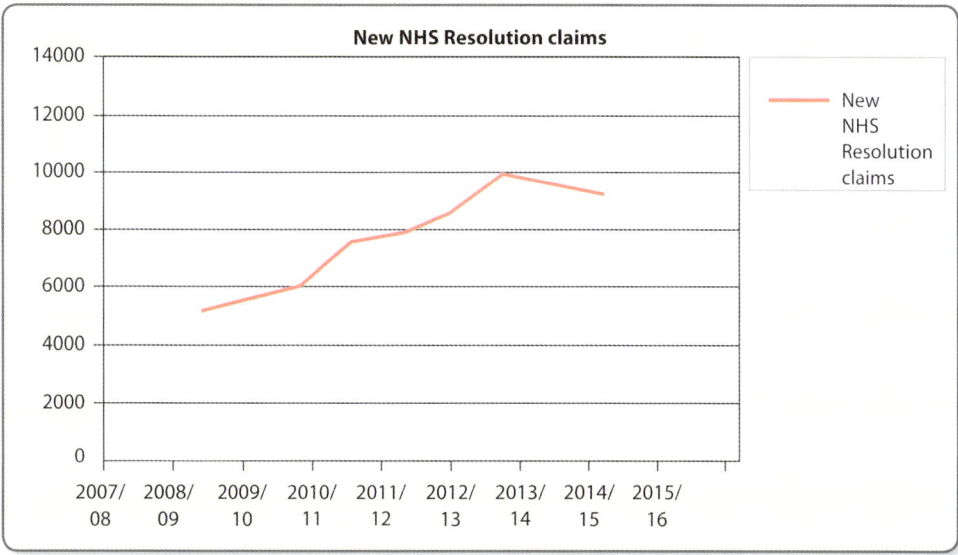

Figure 2.1 New NHS Resolution claims.
Source: NHSLA Annual Reports.

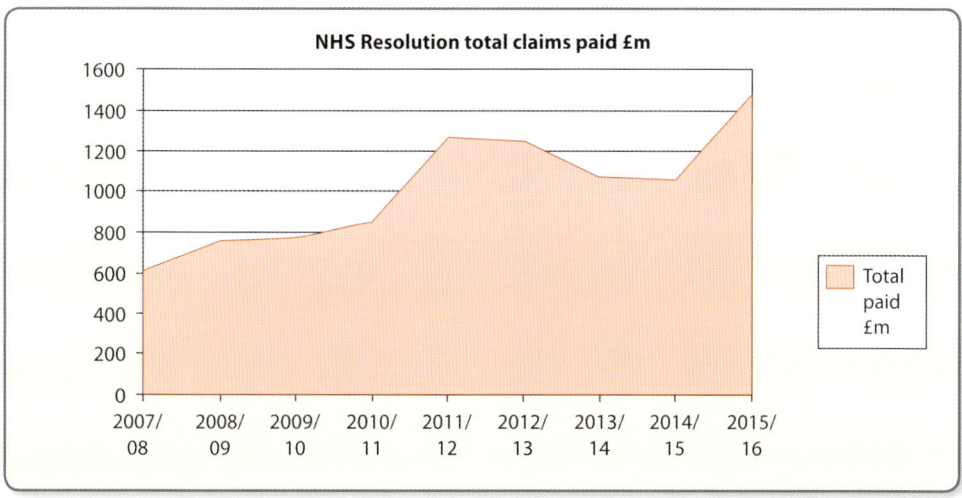

Figure 2.2 Total claims costs for NHS Resolution.
Source: NHSLA Annual Reports.

What happens, if you are sued?

The first inkling of medical litigation normally comes in the form of a solicitor's letter, which includes a request for a copy of the patient medical records. Hospitals and doctors are obliged to provide a copy of the medical records, subject to a suitable release form signed by the patient. A nominal charge can be made for the photocopying.

Normally, the claim must be brought within a set time period, known as "Limitation". This is usually either three years from the time at which the incident occurred, or three years from the time at which the claimant realized that possible negligence may have occurred.

There is no limitation period for medical negligence cases involving children. In people who are mentally incapacitated, the limitation time period is 3 years after the point at which that individual has fully recovered his or her mental capacity.

In England and Wales, this will trigger the Pre-Action Protocol, which was introduced in 1999 to streamline the legal process. This Pre-Action Protocol provides an opportunity to resolve claims before expensive legal proceedings are instigated. In the rest of the United Kingdom, there is no Pre-Action Protocol.

In due course, the solicitor for the complaining patient (known as the claimant) will issue a Letter of Notice, which informs the defendant hospital and/or doctors that legal proceedings are likely to commence. The claimant's solicitor will normally instruct one or more specialists to produce expert medical reports. Expert reports must be impartial, as they are addressed to the court. Many of the cases will proceed no further after the claimant's expert report, as the claimant's expert witness may find no evidence of clinical negligence.

In order to have a successful claim, the claimant's case must meet all of the following three criteria:
1. The defendant (a hospital and/or individual clinicians) owed the patient a duty of care.
2. There was a breach in that duty of care, such that the care provided was below a reasonable standard, which would be expected of a group of competent practitioners, skilled, and experienced in that particular specialty.
3. The breach of duty led to harm or loss for the claimant. The burden of proof in this respect is the "balance of probabilities", which means that there is more than a 50% chance of the harm being caused by the alleged breach of duty.

If the claimant's expert report is supportive of his/her claim, the claimant's solicitor will instigate formal legal proceedings with a formal Letter of Claim. This outlines the legal case, normally incorporating supportive information from the claimant's expert report. This will state the alleged breach of duty (also known as liability) and the subsequent harm or loss (known as causation).

In law, compensation (known as damages) is paid in successful cases, in order to restore the claimant to the situation prior to the negligence. The damages award is split into two parts:
1. General damages, awarded for pain, suffering and loss of amenity.
2. Special damages, which reflect loss of earnings, care costs, pension losses, special equipment or adaptations in the home following the negligence.

Once formal notice of legal proceedings is given, the defendant is given 4 months to investigate and prepare a formal Letter of Response. During this time, the defendant's legal team will instruct its own expert witnesses to provide independent impartial reports.

In the formal Letter of Response, the defendant has three courses of action:
1. Deny the claim entirely
2. Admit some parts of the claim, but deny the remaining allegations
3. Accept liability with an offer to settle.

If it has been decided to deny the allegations and to defend the claim (either in part or in full), the claimant has a further 4 months to issue a Claim Form to the Court together with the original Letter of Claim, Particulars of Claim (setting out the allegations of negligence) and the Schedule of Damages (outlining the financial losses suffered by the claimant). The formal defence must be served within 28 days of the Claim Form, although an extension is often granted to the defendant.

After this, there will be an exchange of reports (known as exchange) and production of documents and information (known as disclosure) between the claimant's and defendant's solicitors.

After exchange and disclosure, there will be a case conference involving a barrister, the legal team for the defendant, the expert witnesses instructed by the defence and the defendant. During the case conference, the defending barrister can assess the merits of the case, and the likelihood of a successful defence at trial.

Following exchange of expert witness evidence, the Wolff Reforms require a joint experts' conference before the case reaches trial. In the conference, the claimant and defence expert witnesses discuss the specific allegations according to a pre-agreed agenda. Some aspects might be agreed by both sides, while there might be continued divergence of opinion about other parts of the case. The aim of the conference is to minimize the time taken in Court, so that the trial focuses solely on the issues, where a difference in opinion remains. The report from the joint experts' conference is submitted to the Court.

Even at this late stage, legal cases are often discontinued after exchange of expert witness evidence and the joint experts' conference. There might be an offer from the defence to settle (sometimes without admission of liability). Alternatively, the claimant may seek to withdraw the claim, if it looks less likely that the claimant might win the case at trial. Some claimants are funded by conditional fee arrangements or their household insurance policies; these will normally only fund the continuation of cases, if the likelihood of a successful claim is greater than 50%.

Ultimately, only 2% of medicolegal cases actually reach the Court for trial.

KEY ASPECTS IN DEFENDING MEDICAL LITIGATION

The legal teams and the Court will try to reconstruct the events, which occurred at the time of the alleged negligence. The case will be judged on the standards of care prevailing at the time of the alleged negligence, and not later on at the time of litigation. The Court will assess whether the care of the claimant was adequate, or whether it fell below what could have been reasonably expected from clinicians skilled in that particular specialty.

The most important aid to defending negligence is the availability of clear and detailed evidence. A major part of this will be the clinical records. Poor record-keeping is a common theme in medicolegal cases, and it is difficult to defend allegations of clinical negligence, when doctors have failed to record their actions during the claimant's care. If something is not written down in the notes, the Court can take the view that it did not happen.

Other forms of evidence include contemporaneous guidelines, which could be local hospital trust documents or national guidance, supportive peer reviewed literature, as well as reports from expert witnesses.

Key witness statements are crucial, particularly from the defending clinician. If a defending clinician decides not to assist the defence legal team (either with a witness statement or appearance in court), it can make the defence case extremely difficult. Knowledgeable input from the defending clinician can also help the defence legal team in ensuring that expert independent reports are instructed from all appropriate specialties required for that particular case.

IMPORTANT LEGAL LANDMARKS

1957 Bolam versus Friern Hospital Management Committee

This ruling sets the traditional standard of care in law. In this case, Mr Bolam underwent electroconvulsive therapy (ECT) for clinical depression in 1954. In the 1950s, there was no universally agreed method to minimize the risk of injuries from the convulsions triggered by the ECT. Mr Bolam was not given any muscle relaxant and he was restrained manually. This was ineffective, and he fractured his pelvis.

The presiding judge, Mr Justice McNair, ruled that the claimant failed to prove his case. He directed the jury by saying:

> *"(A doctor) is not guilty of negligence if he has acted in accordance with the practice accepted as proper by a responsible body of medical men skilled in that particular art... putting it the other way round, a man is not negligent, if he is acting in accordance with such a practice, merely because there is a body of opinion which would take a contrary view."*

This means that the case is defensible, if there would have been a reasonable body of practitioners, who would have acted in the same manner at that time. A reasonable body can be a minority group of doctors, as long as there is suitable and reasonable evidence to support that opinion.

1997 Bolitho versus City and Hackney Health Authority

In this case, a 2-year-old child, Patrick Bolitho was admitted with croup. Twice he went pale with noisy breathing, but recovered spontaneously. The pediatric senior registrar did not attend the child. Shortly afterwards, the child deteriorated rapidly and had a cardiac arrest. He suffered catastrophic brain damage.

It was agreed that the pediatric senior registrar failed in her duty, as she did not attend the child. However, the causation hinged on, whether a pediatrician would have intubated the child after the two episodes of respiratory distress, prior to the cardiac arrest. The pediatric senior registrar said that she would not have intubated the child after the first or second episodes.

Five expert witnesses for the claimant said that any competent doctor would have intubated the child after the first or second episode. The defence argued that there were no signs of progressive respiratory collapse, which might justify the invasive procedure of intubation.

In the trial, although the pediatric senior registrar failed in her duty of care, the judge agreed with the defence that a reasonable (as per Bolam) and *logical* body of expert opinion would not have intubated the child. Hence, the case failed on causation.

> *"The court has to be satisfied that the exponent of the body of opinion relied upon can demonstrate that such opinion has a logical basis. In particular, in cases involving, as they so often do, the weighing of risk against benefits, the judge before accepting a body of opinion as being responsible, reasonable or respectable, will need to be satisfied that, informing their views, the experts have directed their minds to the question of comparative risk and benefits and have reached a defensible conclusion on the matter."*

The Bolitho case is a refinement of the Bolam principles. The judgment from the presiding judge, Lord Browne-Wilkinson, not only required the experts to provide reasonable opinions, but that the reasoning should also withstand logical analysis in order for the judge to view this as being reasonable or responsible.

1986 Gillick versus West Norfolk and Wisbech Area Health Authority

This case arose, as Victoria Gillick, a mother of five young daughters, attempted to get a ruling to say that it would be unlawful for a doctor to prescribe oral contraceptive pills to a young girl under the age of 16 without the knowledge or consent of her parents.

Lord Fraser, the presiding judge, refused Mrs Gillick's application and said the following:

"It seems to me verging on the absurd to suggest that a girl or a boy aged 15 could not effectively consent, for example, to have a medical examination of some trivial injury to his body or even to have a broken arm set. Of course the consent of the parents should normally be asked, but they may not be immediately available. Providing the patient, whether a boy or a girl, is capable of understanding what is proposed, and of expressing his or her own wishes, I see no good reason for holding that he or she lacks the capacity to express them validly and effectively and to authorize the medical man to make the examination or give the treatment which he advises."

Importantly, while the Gillick ruling allows children under the age of 16 to provide valid consent, providing that the child has adequate understanding and intelligence to make up his/her own mind, it does not mean that children under the age of 16 have a right to refuse treatment.

2015 Montgomery versus Lanarkshire Health Board

This landmark case on consent concerned a young diabetic expectant mother, Mrs Montgomery. Diabetic mothers are more likely to have large babies with an increased risk of obstructed labor during normal vaginal delivery. The attending obstetrician's routine policy was not to inform or advise diabetic women about the increased risk of shoulder dystocia, as the doctor felt that the risks of a Cesarean section of the mother outweighed the risks to the baby. Unfortunately, Mrs Montgomery experienced an obstructed labor, and her child was brain-damaged. She was awarded £5.25 million in damages.

The presiding judges, Lord Kerr and Lord Reid, said the following in their judgment:

"An adult of sound mind is entitled to decide which, if any, of the available treatments to undergo, and consent must be obtained before treatment interfering with her bodily integrity is undertaken. The doctor is under a duty to take reasonable care to ensure that the patient is aware of any material risk involved proposed treatment, and of reasonable alternatives. A risk is 'material' if a reasonable person in the patient's position would be likely to attach significance to it, or if the doctor's or should reasonably be aware that their patient would be likely to attach significance to it. Three further points emerge: first, assessing the significance of the risk is fact sensitive and cannot be reduced to percentages. Second, in order to advise, the doctor must engage in dialogue with her patient. Third, the therapeutic exception is limited, and should not be abused."

Table 2.1: Increase in General Medical Council (GMC) referrals over 20 years.

Year	No of registered medical practitioners (RMP)	Enquiries/complaints to GMC (% of RMP)	Likelihood of GMC complaint in 35-year medical career
1992	143,224	1,300 (0.9%)	31.5%
2002	221,250	3,943 (1.8%)	63.0%
2012	252,566	10,347 (4.1%)	143.5%

Column 3: Likelihood of GMC complaint over 35-year career is illustrative only and assumes constant rate of referral.
Source: GMC Annual Reports.

This new test of consent is a significant move away from the test of what a reasonable doctor would recommend to that of what a reasonable patient might choose. It means that a doctor must discuss all treatment options with the patient, when seeking consent for treatment or procedure. There must be dialogue between the doctor and patient, which is comprehensible to the patient. The risks and benefits should be explained clearly to the patient, including any "material risk", which is pertinent and may affect patient outcome.

REFERRAL TO THE GENERAL MEDICAL COUNCIL

Over the last two decades, there has been a very significant increase in referrals of doctors to the GMC, in line with the inexorable rise in medical litigation **(Table 2.1)**. In recent years, there has been a 20% year on year increase in referral rate to the GMC. Similar trends are seen elsewhere, for instance in the USA, Belgium, and Denmark. This accounts in part for the significant rises in the cost of the annual retention fee payable to the GMC.

The most common reasons for GMC referral are listed below in order of frequency:
- Poor clinical care
- Inappropriate relationships with patients
- Concerns about probity
- Working with colleagues
- Other causes.

The most usual source of GMC referral is the employing NHS hospital, followed closely by patients, issues raised through performance monitoring and appraisals, and sometimes the Police.

All surgical specialties have seen an increased referral rate to the GMC. The largest proportional rises have been seen in cardiothoracic, oral maxillofacial surgery, and neurosurgery, with the smallest increases seen in trauma and orthopaedics and plastic surgery **(Figure 2.3)**. In absolute numbers, the greatest number of referrals comes from general surgery and trauma and orthopaedics, as these are the two largest surgical specialties.

IMPLICATIONS OF A COMPLAINT TO THE GENERAL MEDICAL COUNCIL

If a doctor is unfortunate enough to receive a letter from the GMC concerning an investigation, the doctor must inform immediately all the places at which he or she works. It is very difficult to move jobs during an investigation, as one is obliged to declare the GMC complaint to any

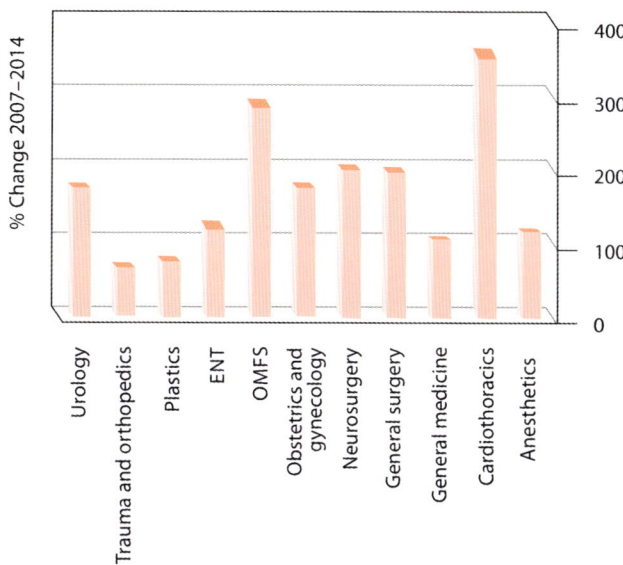

Figure 2.3 Increase in GMC Referrals by Specialty 2007–2014.
% increase compared to 2007 baseline
Source: GMC personal communication

prospective employer. The GMC undertakes to complete the majority of fitness to practice (FTP) cases within 15 months, although some may take significantly longer than this.

The GMC assigns two case examiners to every GMC investigation of allegations against the doctor. The options available to the case examiners are:
- Conclude the case with no further action
- Conclude the case with advice
- Issue a warning to the doctor
- Agree undertakings with the doctors
- Refer the case to a FTP panel hearing.

While the majority of GMC investigations result in the allegations being dropped, the more serious cases are referred to the Medical Practitioners Tribunal Service (MPTS). The MPTS functions independently of the GMC and holds its hearings in Manchester.

If a doctor is referred to the MPTS, the doctor is entitled to be represented by his or her own legal team. The GMC has its own legal team as well as an in-house barrister prosecuting the allegations. As a result, a doctor referred to the MPTS is more likely to be acquitted of the charges, if the defending doctor can engage a legal team including a barrister. The defence fees can be very substantial. The traditional MDOs are usually very supportive of member doctors referred to the MPTS, and normally instruct a legal team and barrister to assist. Some of the newer "Claims Made" medical indemnity insurers may not provide such cover.

If the defending doctor is a consultant, he or she is unable to apply for local Clinical Excellence Awards or for National Awards, while a GMC investigation is pending. Consultants may also experience a drop or loss of private practice income during this time.

If the investigating GMC team regards the allegations as potentially serious, the defending doctor is referred to the MPTS for a tribunal hearing. The first tier of tribunals is the Interim

Orders Panel (IOP). The IOP may decide to place certain restrictions in practice on doctors following the hearing, which must then be notified to all employing hospitals and places at which the doctor works. The IOP restrictions are always reviewed at subsequent hearings, usually at a full FTP tribunal.

An FTP panel has a legal officer and three presiding members, including at least one doctor and at least one layperson. The tribunal hearings are conducted in a similar way to High Court hearings, although the legal protocol is not as well defined as the Civil Court rules.

If allegations are found proven against a doctor, the FTP tribunal will have to consider— (a) how this affects the individual's ability to discharge the duties of a doctor, (b) whether the doctor has reflected upon and recognized the failings, and (c) whether the doctor poses a future risk to patients. If a doctor is found guilty of certain allegations, conditions can be attached to his or her registration, or the doctor may be suspended or erased from the Medical Register.

AVOIDING MEDICAL LITIGATION OR REFERRAL TO THE GENERAL MEDICAL COUNCIL

The most common theme surrounding medical litigation and referrals to the GMC involves poor communication with the patient and family (particularly, if the patient has died as a result of the medical incident). Some patients and their families are prepared to accept medical failings, if a suitable apology is given, and if a thorough investigation has been undertaken with appropriate action to prevent a similar event in the future.

Poor record-keeping can make it very difficult to defend litigation against doctors. Some doctors fail or refuse to write something on a daily basis for patients under their care. This problem can be seen in the private sector as well as in NHS hospitals. In cases, which come to trial or a tribunal, the general adage is "*if it is not written down, it did not happen*".

Keeping full and proper records of discussions is very important, particularly in terms of consent following the recent Montgomery versus Lanarkshire Health Board ruling in 2015. It is crucial that doctors seeking consent of patients document that all options have been discussed and that the material risks of treatment have been explained to the patient.

Of course, good record-keeping and communication takes time. Hence, doctors must manage their time sensibly. This is particularly true in elective work, ensuring that clinics and theatre lists are not overbooked.

Poor clinical performance is the most common reason for referral of a doctor to the GMC by an employing hospital. Doctors must be aware of their duty to audit their performance and to reflect on any incidents. Failure to engage properly with clinical governance can mean that less well-performing doctors can be identified as being outliers and unwilling to improve outcomes by changing clinical practice.

Team working is well recognised as an important part of good patient care. All doctors should remember that their duty to patients over-rides any personal differences that one might have with colleagues. Failure to get on with colleagues is a potent cause of referral to the GMC.

Listening to patients and colleagues is a necessary skill. The pressure of work and personal pride can sometimes make this difficult. However, warning signs about individual patients, the doctor's performance and relationship with colleagues are often raised on a number of occasions prior to litigation or GMC referral. Responding to patient or colleague concerns early will avert complaints, poor patient outcomes, and allegations of negligence.

Key points for clinical practice

- The number of medicolegal cases reported to NHS Resolution increases by over 10% per year, and the number of complaints made to the GMC increases by 20% per year.
- Only 2% of medicolegal cases proceed to trial.
- Most doctors will be involved in medical litigation or a GMC investigation during their career.
- Appropriate medical indemnity is essential and a statutory requirement but terms and cover can vary significantly between traditional MDOs and newer insurance products.
- Good record-keeping is essential, if cases are to be defended successfully.
- The 2015 Montgomery versus Lanarkshire Health Board ruling reinforces the need for good record-keeping, in particular with reference to outlining all suitable treatment options and "material risks" during consent for treatment.
- GMC referrals most commonly relate to concerns about patient care and may be made by the employing hospital, colleagues, or patients.
- The risk of medical litigation can be reduced by good communication, team working, proper recording in the medical notes, and listening to patients and colleagues.
- Good time management allows proper record keeping and helps with patient communication.

BIBLIOGRAPHY

1. Archer J, Regan De Bere S, Bryce M, et al. Understanding the rise in Fitness to Practice Complaints from members of the public. Plymouth: CAMERA (Collaboration for the Advancement of Medical Education Research and Assessment); 2014. pp. 1-161.
2. Elawresources (UK). Bolam v Friern Hospital Management Committee (1957) 1 WLR 583.
3. Elawresources (UK). Bolitho v City and Hackney Health Authority (1957) 4 All ER 771.
4. General Medical Council. Duties of a Doctor. London: General Medical Council; 2013.
5. General Medical Council. Fitness to Practice Annual Statistics Report 2014. London: General Medical Council; 2015.
6. General Medical Council. GMC Thresholds. London: General Medical Council; 2014.
7. General Medical Council. Personal Communication. London: General Medical Council; 2014.
8. GfK NOP Social Research. Research into Fitness to Practice referrals. London: General Medical Council; 2011.
9. Human and Constitutional Rights Resource. Gillick v West Norfolk and Wisbech Area Health Authority (1985) UKHL 7.
10. Medical Protection Society. By your side through change—Strategic Report 2015. London: Medical Protection Society Ltd.; 2016. pp. 1-76.
11. Ministry of Justice. Pre-Action Protocol for the Resolution of Clinical Disputes. London: Ministry of Justice; 2017.
12. NHS Litigation Authority. Annual Report and Accounts 2015 -16 (Presented to Parliament). London: The Stationery Office; 2016.
13. Parliament Health Select Committee. 2012 Accountability Hearing with the General Medical Council. London: The Stationery Office; 2012.
14. Plymouth University Peninsular Schools of Medicine and Dentistry.
15. The General Medical Council. Licence to Practice and Revalidation (Amendment). Regulations Order of Counsel.# London: General Medical Council; 2015.
16. The National Health Service Litigation Authority. Report and Accounts 2011 -12 (Presented to Parliament). London: The Stationery Office; 2012.
17. UK Supreme Court Blog. [2015]. Montgomery v Lanarkshire Health Board (2015) UKSC 11. [online] Available from http://ukscblog.com/case-comment-montgomery-v-lanarkshire-health-board-2015-uksc-11/. [Accessed September, 2017].
18. Williams H, Lees C, Boyd M. The General Medical Council: Fit to Practice? Civitas: Institute for the Study of Civil Society—Doctors' Policy Research Group; 2014.

Section 2

Training in Surgery

CHAPTER

3. Acquisition of Surgical Skills—from Novice to Master; a Fresh Perspective

Chapter 3

Acquisition of surgical skills—from novice to master; a fresh perspective

Sotiris Papaspyros, Joshil V Lodhia, David J O'Regan

INTRODUCTION

The surgical training environment is changing dramatically. Good knowledge, skill, attitude, and behaviors are key ingredients. We can impart, direct, and assess knowledge and skill, hire attitude, and coach behaviors. For surgeons, the critical ingredient is skill and this needs to be both taught and acquired. The outcomes of surgery are directly commensurate with mastery of specific motor skills.[1] Advancement in surgery requires the trainee (and the trainer) to master many skills including open, laparoscopic, endoscopic, and now robotic techniques. These have to be attained in a shorter period of time with legislation that limits the hours of work for the training surgeon. Furthermore, it is no longer acceptable to "practice on the patient" (Professor Sir Barry Jackson, President of the Royal College of Surgeons of England 1998-2001).

In the current era, surgical training has evolved in order to conform to certain conditions— The European Working Time Directive (shorter workweek for residents), increasing complexity of cases and emphasis on operating room efficiency, as well as mitigating medical error, constitute limitations in the preparation of trainees for the operating room experience.

SIMULATION

Simulation techniques are based on established theories of motor skill acquisition and development of expertise.[2] Fitts and Posner's three-stage theory is widely accepted.[3] The three stages or phases of learning are:
- *Stage 1—cognitive*: This stage is characterized by the learner trying to deconstruct the task to be completed. Movements are slow and deliberate.
- *Stage 2—associative*: This stage is when the task is performed with more economy of movement and some parts may become more automatic.
- *Stage 3—autonomous*: This is the stage of unconscious or automatic expertise. Movements are fluent and precise.

It may be difficult to teach in these stages because many expert surgeons have forgotten the deconstruction of their movements through years of "*autonomous*" practice and tasks have become almost automatic. For example, one of the simplest surgical tasks is suturing. However, this can be deconstructed into several parts—the rotation of a needle through tissue can only be effected cleanly, if the alignment of the needle on the needle holder is corrected for the height of the table, surgeon and patient body habitus, and depth of the wound. Needles are made on the circumference of a circle and therefore the needle needs to align 90° across what is to be stitched and 90° into the tissue. 90° is important, as it is a fourth part of a circle and a perfect angle. Rotation of the needle can then happen with understanding of the axis of rotation of the forearm through pronation and supination. The shoulder joint, because of circumduction, enables this to occur in each and every position. This is evident to most people who have taken a screwdriver to build a flat pack cupboard. The cognitive or verbal part of this theory is rarely described by the trainer surgeon, as the task of inserting a suture will only take a second or two.

While simulation models may be useful, they rarely take into account the complexities of surgical practice. It is common to see WETLabs set up with the candidates operating on "organs" at a table while sitting on fixed chairs. No surgeon sits at a table on a fixed chair with the hand, wrist, and elbow working at the same level. Even when a surgeon does sit, they are on mobile stools that have height adjustment capability.

The "correctness" of the handling and movement of surgical instruments is rarely reinforced but are vital to achieving the smooth and reliable performance of the *associative* phase of the Fitts and Posner's model. The acquisition of skills through the three phases of the Fitts and Posner's model does need to be overseen by an expert who can explain and deconstruct the movements in a task. Simulation exercises need to reinforce and build on the correct basic movements and build in complexity. The model should offer immediate feedback of correct and incorrect movement to ensure that the practice of the skill is deliberate. These principles are applied ubiquitously in the world of sports where the field is awash with professional coaches.

The trainee recognizes the need for, and benefit of, simulation.[4,5] The digital era has enabled technology and the profession to respond to this demand. There is also an ever increasing complexity required to simulate the surgical environment. This is recognized to include decision making, team working, understanding of surgical anatomy, and the haptics of movement. Simulated theaters, cadavers, virtual reality, 3D visualization, computer simulation, and NOTSS (nontechnical skills in surgery) are all making significant contributions, but each have their limitations with regards to availability, cost, and efficacy.[6]

High-fidelity simulators offer haptic feedback. It is possible to quantify dexterity, measure time, and record errors as surrogate markers of competency of skills. Laparoscopic surgery has had an advantage over open surgery, as all this information is already digitally recorded and available for analysis.[7,8] Unfortunately, many of these high-fidelity simulators, although very useful for such measurements and research, are often behind "locked doors" for safety and security and therefore not used as frequently as required or intended.

Boot camps are becoming popular and are considered very useful for outlining the principles or surgical skills. The Royal College of Surgeons of Ireland is leading the way in making this compulsory for all surgical trainees. They are supporting this learning with a comprehensive online platform and mobile application.

Deliberate practice affording goal-directed learning and feedback does show better skill enhancement but these are described for high-fidelity models.[9] What is lacking in surgical training are readily available low-fidelity models, which offer feedback that focuses on the correctness of the movement and lightness of touch and which can be used at home.[10]

TECHNICAL SURGICAL SKILL

The key ingredients to any technical surgical skill, whether it is for open, laparoscopic, endoscopic, or robotic surgery, are:

- *"Economy of movement"*—smooth operations are quick operations and quick operations are smooth. This has very little to do with speed but everything to do with effective and efficient movement. Good operators demonstrate a smooth symphony of movement of their hands in concert with the surgical team. This can be seen by the expert surgeon and appreciated by the nontechnical observer.[1] This skill is correlated with long- and short-term outcomes. It is the movement that leads to the outcome (Dubowski).
- *"Lightness of touch"*—this alludes to the respect of the tissue and the proprioceptive feedback from instruments held by the operating surgeon who understands the use of the instrument and is handling it correctly. This is the key message of instructors in golf and the art of the Samurai sword.

This requires mastery, and practice does make perfect.

> *"The more I practice, the luckier I get"*
> Gary Player—three-time USA Golf Masters winner

The 10,000 hours model of skills acquisition does apply to surgery but cannot be achieved in the operating theater alone or with high-fidelity simulation. Trainees need to acquire surgical skill outside the operating theater and these skills do need to be practiced regularly. Moreover, the training of surgical skills needs to focus on the "correctness" and "ergonomics of movement". It needs to be deliberate.[11] Mastery learning requires cognitive interaction, feedback, and repetition over a longer period of time.[6]

Mastery learning is relevant to competency-based learning—it offers prescribed iterative targets that build on principles and complexity. Mastery avoids prescribing the length of time which it requires to obtain a skill. It focuses on "correctness" and encourages "self-awareness" and development. It does require the right mental attitudes—a mindset that focuses on proficiency rather than numbers. These are the principles of martial arts. It is said the difference between a black belt in martial arts and a beginner is attitude and hours of practice. This is the key difference between hours in theater and volume, as opposed to deliberate practice that is recognized amongst experts in sport.[11] There is a very attractive meritocratic and egalitarian attribute to Ericsson's view that everyone can attain expert level of performance with enough hard work, coaching, and feedback. Antagonists have commented that the deliberate practice theory requires "a blindness to ordinary experience" and to the fact that most people who want to become experts—in music, sports, or other domains—do not make it.[12] Furthermore, the literature provides support for Ericsson's contention that many professionals probably never attain true expertise.[2] A recent meta-analysis concluded that the volume of deliberate practice, although unquestionably important as a predictor of individual differences in performance, is not as important as Ericsson and colleagues have argued. In fact, it could only explain up to 30% of the variances.[13]

ATTAINMENT OF TECHNICAL SKILLS

Some surgical practices have developed this concept further with the advent of "entrustable professional activities (EPAs)".[14] The attainment and demonstration of competency thus allow the trainee to then gain experience through volume.

Technical surgery is a motor skill that has to be learnt through practice,[15] but numbers are poor surrogates for competency. "Johnny cannot operate"[16] perhaps because the "why" of what he is doing has not been explained, nor corrected and neither does he have a framework of understanding the movement. The acquisition of motor skills and the principles are well documented, especially in sport. The theory and practice of coaching all athletes at every level involves an understanding of the fundamentals of movement and ergonomics.

Many consultants of today learnt their skills through volume by "practicing" on patients. Basic surgical skills were acquired and rarely taught. Many a trainer, when asked how they execute a specific task will not be able to deconstruct the actions into set up, posture, instrument handling, angles, etc. However, they will, when it is explained be able to make the tacit explicit. The handling of instruments and the passage of the needle through the tissue can be explained in a similar way—this theory has been published and the success of this teaching is realized over 16 years delivering critically acclaimed courses—PAR Excellence and PAR Aorta courses.[10] The feedback from trainees includes *"I wish I was taught this earlier!"* and *"why has not anyone explained this to me before?"*

Most models suggest that the earlier stages should take place outside the operating room. Fidelity may be less important at relatively junior levels of training. Initial acquisition of skills requires block practice, i.e. repetition. This can be done at home on low-fidelity models that offer visible and tactile feedback.

Deliberate practice is the engagement in structured activities created specifically to improve performance in a domain and requires feedback. Are experts "born" or "made"?[17] This is a highly controversial issue. The 10,000 hours needed to become an expert can be helped in the early stages of training with deliberate practice and observation by a skilled trainer.[11]

CONCEPT OF "DIASTOLIC" LEARNING

The cardiac cycle consists of two distinct time periods—(1) systole (contraction of myocardium) and (2) diastole (relaxation of myocardium). Systole is a fixed and relatively short-time period, whereas diastole is longer and varies in length of time depending on hemodynamic conditions. We propose that the surgical skill of suturing any structure (i.e. vein, artery, skin, and subcutaneous tissue) can also be divided in two distinct time periods—(1) the passing of the needle through the structure (systole) and (2) the setting up of the needle on the needle holder in preparation for the next pass (diastole). The above parallelism is elaborated below.

The time it takes an expert surgeon and a trainee to deliver a needle through the tissue is the same for a single pass *"systole"*—but the difference between the expert and the trainees becomes obvious when examining the time it takes to set up to take the second stitch *"diastole"*. The diastolic time is reliant on the ergonomics of the setup, posture, positioning, and handling of the instruments—these skills are tacit for the expert surgeon and have been honed by volume and time. For the trainee, this aspect can be explained and taught.

Have you ever wondered why a good operation appears as smooth? It is because the diastolic period is minimized and the surgeon makes it look easy because they have attended to the setup, their posture, address to the table and angles, i.e. all the negative-passive behaviors. These are sometimes poorly explained, taught, or realized by the trainee or trainer alike but can be understood and more importantly practiced and rehearsed on low-fidelity systems at home.

MARTIAL ARTS

Training in both martial arts and surgery shares common traits. Trainees in both art forms require motivation, dedication, and discipline. Inherent in the ethos of both these sciences is self-improvement, teaching others, and the development of the art form itself. Training in surgery starts during medical school, while for most martial art practitioners, it begins in their first decade of life. It must be highlighted that the Royal Colleges of Surgeons do play an important role in encouraging surgical interest earlier in school and undergraduate students. This early training in surgery is often seen as limited by career hurdles such as entry and passing through medical school, as well as core and higher surgical training. Despite the differences, both art forms have practical elements, which can be deconstructed into smaller segments. Both disciplines take many years of practice before attaining a level of mastery. Given these similarities there are surely aspects of training in martial arts that could be relevant to training in surgery.

Most martial art forms have some defined number basic moves (blocks, footwork, and strikes). On this, "sensei" (the term used for a martial arts instructor) builds a simulated scenario where one practitioner presents the other with a strike or combination of strikes and the other has to carry out a set of defense moves and counter-strikes. These simulations allow novice trainees to develop an appreciation for distancing between the opponent and how each block or strike works. More advanced practitioners experiment with the set technique to appreciate what modifications allow for the most efficient use of energy through positioning and movement. This has an element of spiral training where one task can be beneficial to a beginner but also later to that same trainee, as they have developed other skills. This is important in surgery, as it is not the movement but the anticipated and predicated movements that differentiate a novice from an expert surgeon[15] and the routine from advanced techniques.[18]

Repetition is key in enabling movement to become disassociated from higher thinking. With repetition in martial arts comes the idea of *"correctness"*. It is imperative when developing a skill to ensure the technique is correct without shortcuts or deviation from the principles of efficient movement. This *"correctness"* is reinforced throughout training; a senior practitioner is required to correct himself on the art form when he notices a deviation. Concepts like speed and power can only be built efficiently, if the fundamental movements are correct. This concept applies to surgical training. The basic movements as discussed include instrument handling, mounting of a needle, rotating a needle in and out of tissues at 90° in the sagittal tissue plane, 90° across the two sides to be sutured and 90° into the tissue. This can be summed up simply as place, point, and rotate. Likewise, with knot tying the emphasis is on the movement of the hands when forming and laying down a knot. It is also important to bed the knot down with traction diametrically across the knot. In surgery, speed is often seen as a surrogate marker, when, in fact, it is the surgeon who is most efficient with their movement, not the one who moves their hands the fastest, that is best. Basic surgical skills can be taught on organic material to mimic soft tissues and reinforce lightness of touch. The authors teach the basics of cardiac surgery on potatoes, bananas, and poached eggs. Each give the operator immediate feedback as the potato is mashed, the banana split, and the egg scrambled. These models highlight rough movement and teach lightness of touch. Correct handling of the instruments and positioning the needles on the instruments enables the needle to do the work and glide through the "tissues" on the arc of a perfect circle with minimal damage to the tissue and without bending of needles. This can only be achieved by teaching correctness of needle positioning, body positioning, and axis of rotation of the wrist and forearm. This is intuitive to the expert surgeon but this tacit knowledge, historically learned by volume, is seldom made explicit.

As with all simulation training, it is important to mimic the scenario to best mirror practice. Thus, it is important when practicing suturing or other surgical skills to be standing, thus the trainee can develop an understanding of how body positioning can help. Trainees should be encouraged to correct and modify their own behavior.

COGNITIVE TRAINING

Cognitive training plays a central role in advanced martial arts practice. Mental rehearsal is used to enhance the timing and effectiveness of a technique. This can aptly be applied to surgery.[19] A surgical procedure can easily be broken down into defined steps. Mental rehearsal will not only allow the practitioner to move smoothly from one to the other, but will also prepare them for certain challenging situations such as how to deal with a common bile duct injury during a laparoscopic cholecystectomy or a challenging vascular anastomosis. Rehearsal can prevent many complications and allow the practitioner to take charge when faced with a complication. For example, when faced with a challenging anastomosis, simple steps to help could be preconditioned. Ensuring optimal lighting patient positioning, optimal use of the assistant, and scrub staff can all make a challenging situation more manageable.

The practice of surgery like all sports requires the application of the same principles. It is important to deconstruct the movements and ergonomics required to achieve the action. It is this understanding and rehearsal of these movements that will cultivate and reinforce motor memory resulting in a reduction in the diastolic time of an operation and a smooth transition between actions.

ASSESSMENT OF TECHNICAL SKILLS

Currently, two types of operative skills assessment are in use—(1) rating scales and (2) motion analysis. We have also used rating scales and despite our research we were not able to identify the software required for reliable video interpretation and scoring of hand movement. Currently, there are no defined relevant, robust measures of outcome that can be directly attributed to the effects of training. Therefore, correlating assessment with future performance is difficult. There is some evidence that objective structured assessment of technical skills (OSATS) do reflect the rating level of surgical residents, but these are recognized as inherently associated with subjectivity and do not necessarily provide an accurate record of surgical competence.[20] Respect for tissue is difficult to assess, whereas time and motion analysis can quantify unnecessary moves. The flow of an operation can be deduced from time analysis focusing on the hesitancy of the training surgeon. We have embarked on research to correlate hand movements, proprioception, and tension/force using our low-fidelity models. The subjective video evidence of the benefits of practice, however, is very compelling.

However, as the reliability and validity of assessment tools is increasing, it is likely that competence-based advancement, rather than time served, will become standard in surgical training.[2] William Halsted supported competence-based advancement. He introduced the residency training system, which remains the cornerstone of surgical training more than a century later.

In our opinion (supported by our experience with the PAR courses over last 16 years), there is compelling evidence that basic surgical skills can reliably be taught and learned using low-fidelity models and deliberate practice. Three of the parameters measured (flow/rhythm, precision, and rotation) are qualitative and subjective by definition. However, time/pace, which was the only objectively quantifiable parameter showed an impressive 30% improvement. Furthermore, participants reported their average practice times, but they were not directly observed. In our experience, character traits such as persistence and motivation play a role on how much time a trainee spends practicing and this has direct implications on their ability to perform the task. This is also reflected in the literature.

CONCLUSION

Acquisition of surgical technical skills is a long and complex process, which can be deconstructed into different stages. Simulation is an important component of modern surgical training programs.[21] Low-fidelity simulation models can reliably be used to achieve significant progress through the early stages of the learning curve. Low-fidelity models can be reliable and are valid to all aspects of surgery at low cost.[22] The literature confirms that surgical expertise is reached through deliberate practice—surgeons are made and not born.[17]

Accurate assessment of an individual's abilities at an early stage may be critical in their choice of career, and whether they have a realistic chance of becoming an expert through deliberate practice. The usefulness of any particular assessment method is determined by its reliability, validity, impact on future learning and practice, acceptability to learners, faculty and costs.[22]

The advantages of mastery of learning are obvious.[6] There are many parallels with sport. We believe the gap in training is to be found at the beginning—it is only by mastering the basics that the aspiring surgeon can progress their skills and benefit from high-fidelity models. We need to look at all the models as part of a spectrum; but at every stage, we need to ensure that the models and practices mirror what we actually do in the operating theater and are embedded in structured education programs.[18]

> **Key points for clinical practice**
> - Surgical skills can be practiced on low-fidelity models.
> - The acquisition of skills follows the three phases of the Fitts-Posner model—cognitive, associative, and autonomous.
> - The phases of learning are deliberate and require models that can be set up and used at home to simulate the skill and offer visible and proprioceptive feedback to the practitioner.
> - The cognitive phase needs to focus on the correctness of the movement.
> - A trainee's practice needs to be overseen by a coach or master of the skills.
> - There are many parallels between training in surgery and sport or martial arts.
> - Mastery is a journey.

REFERENCES

1. Birkmeyer JD, Finks JF, O'Reilly A, et al. Surgical skill and complication rates after bariatric surgery. N Engl J Med. 2013;369(15):1434-42.
2. Reznick RK, MacRae H. Teaching surgical skills--changes in the wind. N Engl J Med. 2006;355(25):2664-9.

3. Fitts PM, Posner MI. Human performance. Belmont, CA: Brooks/Cole; 1967.
4. Boyd KB, Olivier J, Salameh JR. Surgical residents' perception of simulation training. Am Surg. 2006;72(6): 521-4.
5. Milburn JA, Khers G, Malone PSC, et al. Introduction, availability and role of simulation in surgical education and training: review of current evidence and recommendations from the Association of Surgeons in Training. Int J Surg. 2012;10(8):393-8.
6. Siddaiah-Subramanya M, Smith S, Lonie J. Mastery learning: how is it helpful? An analytical review. Adv Med Educ Pract. 2017;8:269-75.
7. Taffinder N, Sutton C, Fishwick RJ, et al. Validation of virtual reality to teach and assess psychomotor skills in laparoscopic surgery: results from randomised controlled studies using the MIST VR laparoscopic simulator. Stud Health Technol Inform. 1998;50:124-30.
8. Uemaura M, Tomikawa M, Kumashiro R, et al. Analysis of hand motion differentiates expert and novice surgeons. J Surg Research. 2014;188(1):8-13.
9. Issenberg SB, McGaghie WC, Petrusa ER, et al. Features and uses of high-fidelity medical simulations that lead to effective learning: a BEME systematic review. Med Teach. 2005;27(1):10-28.
10. Papaspyros SC, Kar A, O'Regan D. Surgical ergonomics. Analysis of technical skills, simulation models and assessment methods. Int J Surg. 2015;18:83-7.
11. Ericsson KA. Deliberate practice and the acquisition and maintenance of expert performance in medicine and related domains. Acad Med. 2004;79 (10 Suppl):S70-S81.
12. Hambrick DZ, Oswald FL, Altmann EM, et al. Deliberate practice: Is that all it takes to become an expert? Intelligence. 2014;45:34-45.
13. Macnamara BN, Hambrick DZ, Oswald FL. Deliberate practice and performance in music games sports education and professions: a meta-analysis. Psychol Sci. 2014;25(8):1608-18.
14. Ten Cate O. Competency-based education; entrustable professional activities, and the power of language. J Grad Med Educ. 2013;5(1):6-7.
15. Dubrowski A, Backstein D. The contributions of Kinesiology to Surgical Education. J Bone Joint Surg. 2004;86A:2778-81.
16. Bell RH Jr. Why Johnny cannot operate. Surgery. 2009;146(4):533-42.
17. Sadideen H, Alnabd A, Saadeddin M, et al. Surgical experts: Born or made? Int J Surg. 2013;11(90):773-8.
18. Maran NJ, Glavin RJ. Low- to high-fidelity simulation—a continuum of medical education? Med Educ. 2003;37(Suppl 1):22-8.
19. Wallace L, Raison N, Ghumman F, et al. Cognitive training: How can it be adapted for surgical education? Surgeon. 2016;15(4):231-9.
20. Hopmans C, den Hoed P, van der Laan L, et al. Assessment of surgery residents' operative skills in the operating theater using modified Objective Structured Assessment of Technical Skills (OSATS): a prospective multicenter study. Surgery. 2014;156(5):1078-88.
21. Sarker SK, Patel B. Simulation in Surgical Training (Review Article). Int J Clin Pract. 2007;61(12):2120-5.
22. Van der Vleuten CP. The assessment of professional competence: developments, research and practical implications. Adv Health Sci Educ. 1996;1(1):41-67.

Section 3

Breast Surgery

CHAPTERS

4. Assessment of Margins in Breast Cancer Surgery
5. Lobular Carcinoma in Situ

Chapter 4

Assessment of margins in breast cancer surgery

Dorin Dumitru, Michael Douek

INTRODUCTION

Breast-conserving surgery (BCS), followed by adjuvant radiotherapy, is the preferred standard treatment for localized early breast cancer, as it has the same long-term survival as mastectomy.[1,2] Successful BCS entails complete excision of the tumor with adequate margins and when margins are involved with tumor, reoperation for re-excision is recommended. Reasons for involved margins and need for reoperation include poor patient selection for BCS, variations in surgical technique, variations in histopathological specimen examination, and definition of margins, inadequate imaging and localization, underestimation of tumor extent and more aggressive cancer. Houssami et al.[3] in a large meta-analysis including 21 studies and 14,571 patients with invasive breast cancer reported that the odds ratio (OR) for local recurrence was significantly increased with positive margins [OR 2.42 (p < 0.001)]. There was no difference in rates of local recurrence between individual margin widths of more than 1, more than 2, or more than 5 mm when models were adjusted for administration of radiotherapy boost and endocrine therapy. An updated meta-analysis[4] including 33 studies and 28,162 patients with invasive breast cancer confirmed that negative margins reduce the odds of local recurrence but that increasing the distance for defining negative margins, was not significantly associated with reduced odds of local recurrence. However, there is international variation on what constitutes an adequate margin. The Society of Surgical Oncology and the American Society for Radiation Oncology published consensus guidelines on margins for BCS, recommending "no tumor on ink"[5] for invasive cancer and 2 mm for ductal carcinoma in situ (DCIS).[6] The European St Gallen International Expert Consensus Conference, adopted the North American recommendation of "no tumor on ink" for invasive disease regardless of tumor biology, and 2 mm for DCIS.[7] In the UK, the Association of Breast Surgery adopted 1 mm, as the minimum margin for both invasive disease and DCIS.[8]

When margins are involved with cancer or DCIS, reoperation for re-excision of margins is recommended and Jeevan et al.[9] in a cohort study including 55,297 women undergoing primary BCS for cancer reported that 20% of women required one or more reoperations for re-excision and that for pure DCIS, the rate was 29.5%. However, since then guidelines for adequate margins have changed, which is recognized to reduce rates of reoperation. Patient selection for BCS depends on the extent of the cancer (unifocal versus multifocal), the size of the tumor relative to the size of the breast, its location and on patient's preference. It is most important to select appropriate patients for BCS in order to reduce reoperation rates. For those patients who require chemotherapy, administering it before surgery reduces re-excision rates from 20.3% to 11.4% (n = 71,627; OR 0.53; p < 0.001). But downsizing of tumors with preoperative chemotherapy is associated with an increase in local recurrence in the long-term. The EBCTCG[10] in a meta-analysis of 4,756 women entered into 10 randomized controlled trials comparing neoadjuvant with adjuvant chemotherapy found that although suitability for BCS was higher with neoadjuvant chemotherapy (65% vs 49%), so was the 15-year local recurrence [21.4% vs 15.9%; rate ratio 1.37 (95% CI 1.17–1.61); p = 0.0001]. It is thus important to consider neoadjuvant chemotherapy in those patients wishing to potentially avoid mastectomy rather than those who are already suitable for BCS at presentation.

The widespread use of breast-screening programs, increased patient awareness, and increased use of advanced imaging modalities [including breast magnetic resonance imaging (MRI)] has increased the identification of clinically occult nonpalpable breast cancers.[11] In the UK, one-third of all breast cancers diagnosed are nonpalpable and even higher rates approaching 50% are observed in other developed countries with widespread breast-screening programs. For nonpalpable breast cancer, both screen detected and resulting from administration of neoadjuvant chemotherapy, BCS requires localization. Reoperation rates for re-excision of margins with wire-guided localization, the most common used technique, are reported to range between 10% and 43% for invasive and in situ disease.

Reoperation following BCS, increases postoperative complications,[12] can delay administration of subsequent adjuvant treatment, affects the cosmetic outcome and has psychological and economic consequences.[13] It is also associated with an increase in local and distant recurrence.[14]

So, involved margins and reoperation for re-excision are important clinical challenges. When trying to avoid need for re-excision, besides the key factors of appropriate patient selection for BCS and for systemic treatment and good pre-operative planning (including localization), there are some techniques for intra-operative assessment although no single technique is internationally recognized as standard of care. The key benefit of these techniques is the timely recognition of margin involvement with sufficient accuracy during surgery, to enable excision of cavity shaves and avoid subsequent reoperation. A systematic review and meta-analysis,[15] compared the diagnostic accuracy of intraoperative techniques for margin assessment and found that cytology (pooled sensitivity 0.91 and pooled specificity 0.95) and frozen section (pooled sensitivity 0.86 and pooled specificity 0.96), are the most accurate techniques. These techniques include several established techniques and some novel techniques.

ESTABLISHED TECHNIQUES FOR INTRAOPERATIVE ASSESSMENT OF MARGINS

Established techniques include routine cavity shaves, frozen section, cytology, intraoperative ultrasound (IOUS), and specimen radiography.

Routine cavity shaves, frozen section, and cytology

It has been recognized for many years that excision of further cavity shaves at the initial surgery and reduces reoperation rate.[16,17] This was confirmed in a randomized controlled trial involving 235 patients with stage 0–III breast cancer undergoing BCS with or without routine cavity shaves.[18] Routine cavity shaves significantly reduced margin positivity rate (19% vs 34%; p = 0.01). This led to a significant reduction in rate of reoperation for re-excision of margins (10% vs 21%; p = 0.02). However, cavity shaves are not usually assessed during surgery. The decision on whether to use frozen section or cytology, rests with the experience of local pathologists and their availability, and given that both are time consuming. In terms of diagnostic accuracy, frozen section was found on meta-analysis[15] to have a pooled sensitivity of 0.86 (95% CI 0.78–0.91) and a specificity of 0.96 (95% CI 0.92–0.98) for the detection of margin involvement. By comparison, cytology had a pooled sensitivity of 0.91 (95% CI 0.71–0.97) and a specificity of 0.95 (95% CI 0.90–0.98). These tissue-based techniques have very poor uptake in routine clinical practice most likely due to logistical issues of slow turnaround times, disruption of operating lists and availability of pathology staff. Use of frozen section is reported to reduce rates of re-operation from 13.2% (nationally) to 3.6% at a single institution using routine frozen section.[19]

Bolger et al.[20] compared three different established intraoperative margin assessment techniques—routine cavity shave margins (n = 70), macroscopic assessment of margins (n = 68), and no formal margin assessment (n = 50). Routine cavity shaves with a minimum thickness of 1 cm were taken from four surfaces and macroscopic assessment of the margins was performed by a pathologist. The distance of tumor from each radial margin (medial, lateral, superior, and inferior) was measured and if less than 5 mm, a cavity shave was excised. The remaining group underwent excision of further cavity shaves at the discretion of the operating surgeon. Comparison with formal histopathological evaluation, revealed a re-excision rate of 25% compared with 34% for the group without formal evaluation of margins and a statistically significant reduction in the chance of residual disease following the initial surgical procedure (p = 0.02). A systematic review and meta-analysis[15] reported a pooled sensitivity for the detection of involved margins of 0.86 [95% confidence interval (95% CI) 0.78–0.91] and pooled specificity of 0.96 (95% CI 0.92–0.98) for frozen section; and for cytology, a pooled sensitivity of 0.91 (95% CI 0.71–0.97) and a pooled specificity of 0.95 (95% CI 0.90–0.98).

Although frozen section[21] and cytology are effective, they are operator dependent, resource intensive, and time consuming. With frozen section, the tissue can be damaged with compression artefacts challenging histological evaluation. Cytology (e.g. touch/imprint/scrape) cannot distinguish invasive from in situ disease, and cannot provide information of margin width.

Intraoperative imaging

Portable ultrasound is now used in a variety of clinical settings including insertion of central lines by anesthetists and is therefore widely available. Although the image quality is lower than departmental ultrasound machines, there are useful indications for portable ultrasound in breast surgery,[22] including IOUS. The Dutch COBALT trial randomized 134 women with palpable early stage primary invasive breast cancer (T1-2, N0-1) to either ultrasound-guided surgery or palpation-guided surgery. IOUS significantly reduced tumor involved margin rate (3% vs 17%; p = 0.0093) and resulted in smaller excision volumes (38 vs 57 cm^3; p = 0.002).[23] In this trial, focally involved excision margins were treated with a radiotherapy boost rather than a reoperation for re-excision. Seven (11%) patients in the IOUS group and 19 (28%) of those who received palpation-guided surgery required additional treatment (17%, 3–30; p = 0.015) for involved margins. A systematic review and meta-analysis[15] reported IOUS had a pooled sensitivity of 0.59 (95% CI 0.36–0.79) and a pooled specificity of 0.81 (95% CI 0.66–0.91) for detection of margin involvement. Despite increased accessibility to ultrasound, the overall performance of ultrasound by breast surgeons remains consistently low. IOUS is operator dependent, requires additional training, and suspicious calcifications are often invisible on ultrasound.

Many surgeons perform intraoperative radiological assessment of impalpable (and often palpable) lesions using portable X-ray devices such as the BioVision (Faxitron Bioptics LLC, Arizona, USA). McCornick et al.[24] found that intraoperative specimen radiography more than halved positive margins rates (12% vs 5%), while Layfield et al.[25] reported that use of intraoperative specimen radiography for palpable breast cancer reduced mean specimen weight and improved cosmesis, without increasing re-excision rates. In a prospective study involving 170 patients with both palpable and impalpable lesions, margin status was assessed systematically with intraoperative specimen radiography, using a dedicated intraoperative X-ray device (Faxitron MX20). Margins were evaluable in 91.2% of cases and were assessed according to the histological subtype. A 10-mm margin on specimen radiograph led to negative margins in 98.5% of invasive ductal carcinomas, 90% of invasive lobular carcinomas, and 78.5% of DCIS cases with an overall margin positivity rate of 6.5% when intraoperative. A systematic review and meta-analysis[15] reported specimen radiography had a pooled sensitivity of 0.53 (95% CI 0.45–0.61) and a pooled specificity of 0.84 (95% CI 0.77–0.89) for the detection of margin involvement. However, specimen radiographs can be performed within the operating room, provide results that are interpretable by the surgeon, and avoid the need for additional personnel.

NOVEL TECHNOLOGIES FOR MARGIN ASSESSMENT

Novel intraoperative margin assessment techniques include imaging, optical techniques, bioimpedance/radiofrequency, and mass spectrometry. Novel imaging techniques to image specimens include microcomputed computed tomography (CT) and high-frequency ultrasound are at a very early stage of development and require access to imaging and interpretation, which are significant drawbacks. The AMIGO study[26] evaluated MRI-guided BCS in specialized operating facilities and is unlikely to become widely available beyond specialist centers.

Following proof of principle of novel technologies, frequently clinical studies are inadequately designed and or are under powered, preventing their clinical application beyond those clinicians evaluating them. Very few of these techniques have been evaluated within adequately powered prospective clinical trials or randomized controlled trials. The later are best suited to provide evidence on a technique's ability to be rapid and practical, its diagnostic accuracy (comparable to established techniques), reduction in reoperation rate, and improved cost-effectiveness. Several techniques with clinical evidence are discussed below.

MarginProbe and ClearEdge

The MarginProbe (Dune Medical Services Limited, Caesarea, Israel) is based on reflection of radiofrequency waves that measure local electrical properties of breast tissue within the radiofrequency range. The device creates an electrical signature of tissues that is dependent on the membrane potential, nuclear morphology, and intercellular contact. The device also takes account of differences in vascularity, and collectively these factors enable distinction between malignant and benign/normal tissue. It has been designed as an adjunct to routine surgical methods, the hand-held device is convenient to use and the probe has a 7-mm footprint, which is employed to take between five and eight measurements from each of the six surfaces of an excised specimen. A positive reading indicates tumor cells present within 1 mm of the resection margin and a cavity shave is then performed. The overall sensitivity for detection of malignancy is 70–100% with specificity of 70–87%.[27] Two randomized controlled trials evaluated MarginProbe to date. Allweis et al.[28] randomized 300 women undergoing BCS to device or no device arms. Reoperation was lower in the device arm compared to the control arm, but the difference was not statistically significant (12.6% vs 18.6%; p = 0.098). Schnabel et al.[29] randomized 596 women with impalpable breast cancer suitable for BCS to device or no device arms. Reoperation rate was lower in the device arm (19.8% vs 25.8%) and the reduction in reoperation rate was significant amongst patients who had positive margins in the main tumor specimen (10% vs 20.8%; p = 0.002).

Another related technology is the ClearEdge (LsBioPath, Saratoga, USA) imaging device, which measures the electrical conductivity and capacitance of the tissue using an array of electrodes with fraction of a millimeter resolution. The 10 × 10 array of tiny electrodes penetrates the edge of the excised tissue (margins) to a default depth of 3 mm with a spatial size of 13 × 13 mm. The device measures 180 spatially resolved locations for each probe location and provides a full tissue image within 3 seconds. The color-coded image indicates both the location and the propagation direction of the picked up tissue abnormality. A preliminary study was conducted in two phases to validate the safety and accuracy of the device ex vivo and then intraoperatively to estimate any reduction in reoperation. A larger prospective trial is now needed for further clinical evaluation.

Optical imaging

Optical imaging utilizes different wavelengths of light either directed onto tissues, emitted from tissues for visualization, or analysis of emitted spectra. Techniques include Terahertz pulsed imaging,[30] Raman spectroscopy, optical coherence tomography, and confocal microscopy. A meta-analysis[15] included the later three techniques and found a pooled sensitivity for the detecting of margin involvement of 0.85 (95% CI 0.74–0.91) and a pooled specificity of 0.87 (95% CI 0.65–0.96). Another technique, Cerenkov luminescence imaging (CLI), combines optical and molecular imaging by detecting light emitted by 18F-FDG, administered to patients intravenously prior to surgery. Its main drawbacks are a short-operating window and radiation exposure.[31]

Intelligent knife

The i-knife (intelligent knife) analyzes the electrosurgical plume of diathermy smoke to determine the structural lipid profile of tissue. This is based on rapid evaporative ionization mass spectrometry (REIMS) with online chemical analysis of the electrosurgical aerosol. Use of electrical diathermy for cutting or coagulation of tissue, triggers a cellular explosion from heat dissipation with release of cellular product into a gas phase. Chemical analysis using both cutting and coagulation modalities have been performed on a normal and tumor breast tissue and validation spectra correlated with tissue microscopic. The i-knife has now been optimized for real-time intraoperative analysis of breast tissue and yields high rates of sensitivity and specificity (sensitivity 90.9% and specificity of 98.8%).[32] REIMS shows promising results for detection of positive resection margins intraoperatively (100%) and has a sensitivity of 77.3%. Clinical evaluation is now required to reliably assess accuracy for intraoperative margin assessment.

CONCLUSION

Involved margins and reoperation for re-excision are important clinical challenges. When trying to avoid need for re-excision, besides the key factors of appropriate patient selection for BCS and for systemic treatment and good preoperative planning (including localization), there are some techniques for intraoperative assessment although no single technique is internationally recognized as standard of care. Techniques for intraoperative assessment of margins include several established techniques and some novel techniques. The most accurate established techniques for intraoperative assessment of margins are cytology and frozen section, but they have very poor uptake in routine clinical practice most likely due to logistical issues of slow turnaround times, disruption of operating lists, and availability of pathology staff. IOUS significantly reduces tumor involved margin rate, results in smaller excision volumes, and reduces need for further treatment (radiotherapy boost or reoperation) for involved margins. Intraoperative radiological assessment of impalpable and palpable tumors is frequently undertaken using portable X-ray devices to perform specimen radiographs, which can be readily interpreted by the surgeon. Of the available novel devices for intraoperative assessment of margins during BCS, only MarginProbe has been evaluated within randomized controlled trials.

> **Key points for clinical practice**
>
> - Reasons for involved margins and need for reoperation include poor patient selection for BCS, variations in surgical technique, variations in histopathological specimen examination and definition of margins, inadequate imaging and localization and underestimation of tumor extent or more aggressive cancer.
> - The Society of Surgical Oncology and the American Society for Radiation Oncology published consensus guidelines on margins for BCS, recommending "no tumor on ink" for invasive cancer and 2 mm for DCIS. The European St Gallen International Expert Consensus Conference adopted the North American recommendation of "no tumor on ink" for invasive disease regardless of tumor biology, and 2 mm for DCIS. In the UK, the association of breast surgery adopted 1 mm as the minimum margin for both invasive disease and DCIS.
> - For those patients, who require chemotherapy, administering it before surgery reduces re-excision rates but downsizing of tumors with preoperative chemotherapy and is associated with an increase in local recurrence in the long-term.
> - The most accurate established techniques for intraoperative assessment of margins are cytology and frozen section, but they are operator dependent, resource intensive, and time consuming.
> - Routine cavity shaves significantly reduce margin positivity rate reoperation for re-excision of margins.
> - Intraoperative ultrasound significantly reduces tumor involved margin rate, results in smaller excision volumes and reduces need for further treatment (radiotherapy boost or reoperation) for involved margins.
> - Intraoperative radiological assessment of impalpable and palpable tumors is frequently undertaken using portable X-ray devices to perform specimen radiographs, which can be readily interpreted by the surgeon.
> - Of the available novel devices for intraoperative assessment of margins during BCS, only MarginProbe has been evaluated within randomized controlled trials.

REFERENCES

1. Veronesi U, Cascinelli N, Mariani L, et al. Twenty-year follow-up of a randomized study comparing breast-conserving surgery with radical mastectomy for early breast cancer. N Engl J Med. 2002;347(16):1227-32.
2. Fisher B, Anderson S, Bryant J, et al. Twenty-year follow-up of a randomized trial comparing total mastectomy, lumpectomy, and lumpectomy plus irradiation for the treatment of invasive breast cancer. N Engl J Med. 2002;347(16):1233-41.
3. Houssami N, Macaskill P, Marinovich ML, et al. Meta-analysis of the impact of surgical margins on local recurrence in women with early-stage invasive breast cancer treated with breast-conserving therapy. Eur J Cancer. 2010;46(18):3219-32.
4. Houssami N, Macaskill P, Marinovich ML, et al. The association of surgical margins and local recurrence in women with early-stage invasive breast cancer treated with breast-conserving therapy: a meta-analysis. Ann Surg Oncol. 2014;21(3):717-30.
5. Moran MS, Schnitt SJ, Giuliano AE, et al. Society of Surgical Oncology-American Society for Radiation Oncology consensus guideline on margins for breast-conserving surgery with whole-breast irradiation in stages I and II invasive breast cancer. Ann Surg Oncol. 2014;21(3):704-16.
6. Morrow M, Van Zee KJ, Solin LJ, et al. Society of Surgical Oncology-American Society for Radiation Oncology-American Society of Clinical Oncology Consensus Guideline on Margins for Breast-Conserving Surgery with Whole-Breast Irradiation in Ductal Carcinoma In Situ. Ann Surg Oncol. 2016;23(12):3801-10.
7. Curigliano G, Burstein HJ, E PW, et al. De-escalating and escalating treatments for early-stage breast cancer: the St. Gallen International Expert Consensus Conference on the Primary Therapy of Early Breast Cancer 2017. Ann Oncol. 2017;28(8):1700-12.
8. Association of Breast Surgery. ABS Consensus Margin Width in Breast Conservation Surgery. 2015.
9. Jeevan R, Cromwell DA, Trivella M, et al. Reoperation rates after breast conserving surgery for breast cancer among women in England: retrospective study of hospital episode statistics. BMJ. 2012;345(345):e4505.
10. Early Breast Cancer Trialists' Collaborative Group (EBCTCG). Long-term outcomes for neoadjuvant versus adjuvant chemotherapy in early breast cancer: meta-analysis of individual patient data from ten randomised trials. Lancet Oncol. 2018;19(1):27-39.
11. Ahmed M, Rubio IT, Klaase JM, et al. Surgical treatment of nonpalpable primary invasive and in situ breast cancer. Nat Rev Clin Oncol. 2015;12(11):645-63.
12. Xue DQ, Qian C, Yang L, et al. Risk factors for surgical site infections after breast surgery: a systematic review and meta-analysis. Eur J Surg Oncol. 2012;38(5):375-81.
13. Al-Ghazal SK, Fallowfield L, Blamey RW. Does cosmetic outcome from treatment of primary breast cancer influence psychosocial morbidity? Eur J Surg Oncol. 1999;25(6):571-3.
14. Kouzminova NB, Aggarwal S, Aggarwal A, et al. Impact of initial surgical margins and residual cancer upon re-excision on outcome of patients with localized breast cancer. Am J Surg. 2009;198(6):771-80.
15. St John ER, Al-Khudairi R, Ashrafian H, et al. Diagnostic Accuracy of Intraoperative Techniques for Margin Assessment in Breast Cancer Surgery: A Meta-analysis. Ann Surg 2017;265(2):300-10.
16. Jacobson AF, Asad J, Boolbol SK, et al. Do additional shaved margins at the time of lumpectomy eliminate the need for re-excision? Am J Surg. 2008;196(4):556-8.
17. Mook J, Klein R, Kobbermann A, et al. Volume of excision and cosmesis with routine cavity shave margins technique. Ann Surg Oncol. 2012;19(3):886-91.
18. Chagpar AB, Killelea BK, Tsangaris TN, et al. A Randomized, Controlled Trial of Cavity Shave Margins in Breast Cancer. N Engl J Med. 2015;373(6):503-10.
19. Boughey JC, Hieken TJ, Jakub JW, et al. Impact of analysis of frozen-section margin on reoperation rates in women undergoing lumpectomy for breast cancer: evaluation of the National Surgical Quality Improvement Program data. Surgery. 2014;156(1):190-7.
20. Bolger JC, Solon JG, Khan SA, et al. A comparison of intra-operative margin management techniques in breast-conserving surgery: a standardised approach reduces the likelihood of residual disease without increasing operative time. Breast Cancer. 2015;22(3):262-8.
21. Osako T, Nishimura R, Nishiyama Y, et al. Efficacy of intraoperative entire-circumferential frozen section analysis of lumpectomy margins during breast-conserving surgery for breast cancer. Int J Clin Oncol. 2015;20(6):1093-101.
22. Ahmed M, Abdullah N, Cawthorn S, et al. Why should breast surgeons use ultrasound? Breast Cancer Res Treat. 2014;145(1):1-4.
23. Krekel NM, Haloua MH, Lopes Cardozo AM, et al. Intraoperative ultrasound guidance for palpable breast cancer excision (COBALT trial): a multicentre, randomised controlled trial. Lancet Oncol. 2013;14(1):48-54.

24. McCormick JT, Keleher AJ, Tikhomirov VB, et al. Analysis of the use of specimen mammography in breast conservation therapy. Am J Surg. 2004;188(4):433-6.
25. Layfield DM, May DJ, Cutress RI, et al. The effect of introducing an in-theatre intraoperative specimen radiography (IOSR) system on the management of palpable breast cancer within a single unit. Breast. 2012;21(4):459-63.
26. Golshan M, Sagara Y, Wexelman B, et al. Pilot study to evaluate feasibility of image-guided breast-conserving therapy in the advanced multimodal image-guided operating (AMIGO) suite. Ann Surg Oncol. 2014;21(10):3356-7.
27. Thill M. MarginProbe: intraoperative margin assessment during breast conserving surgery by using radiofrequency spectroscopy. Expert Rev Med Devices. 2013;10(3):301-15.
28. Allweis TM, Kaufman Z, Lelcuk S, et al. A prospective, randomized, controlled, multicenter study of a real-time, intraoperative probe for positive margin detection in breast-conserving surgery. Am J Surg. 2008;196(4):483-9.
29. Schnabel F, Boolbol SK, Gittleman M, et al. A randomized prospective study of lumpectomy margin assessment with use of MarginProbe in patients with nonpalpable breast malignancies. Ann Surg Oncol. 2014;21(5):1589-95.
30. Grootendorst MR, Fitzgerald AJ, Brouwer de Koning SG, et al. Use of a handheld terahertz pulsed imaging device to differentiate benign and malignant breast tissue. Biomed Opt Express. 2017;8(6):2932-45.
31. Grootendorst MR, Cariati M, Pinder SE, et al. Intraoperative Assessment of Tumor Resection Margins in Breast-Conserving Surgery Using (18)F-FDG Cerenkov Luminescence Imaging: A First-in-Human Feasibility Study. J Nucl Med. 2017;58(6):891-8.
32. St John ER, Balog J, McKenzie JS, et al. Rapid evaporative ionisation mass spectrometry of electrosurgical vapours for the identification of breast pathology: towards an intelligent knife for breast cancer surgery. Breast Cancer Res. 2017;19(1):59.

Chapter 5

Lobular carcinoma in situ

Kalnisha Naidoo, Sarah E Pinder

INTRODUCTION

Lobular neoplasia (LN), also referred to as in situ lobular neoplasia, is an umbrella term encompassing atypical lobular hyperplasia (ALH) and lobular carcinoma in situ (LCIS) and is a process arising in the terminal duct lobular unit (TDLU) of the breast.[1,2] Characteristically, in the classical form, both comprise a relatively uniform population of discohesive, rounded cells.[2,3] In fact, the distinction between ALH and LCIS lies not in cellular composition, but rather in the extent of disease; if less than 50% of the acini in a TDLU are expanded by such cells, the condition is classified as ALH, with greater involvement being termed LCIS.[2-4] Although both these entities form part of the same disease spectrum, the distinction between the two is considered relevant because the relative risk of malignancy associated with LCIS is approximately twice as high as that for ALH, which in turn carries a risk that is 4–5 times higher than that of the general population.[4-7] Thus, it would seem appropriate that whether, and how to, screen for, as well as how to sample and manage these lesions should reflect this "continuum of risk". There is limited data on the clinical behavior of more recently recognized, but uncommon, entities such as pleomorphic LCIS and classical LCIS with necrosis but these, biologically, are likely to behave differently to the more common classical forms of the disease.

DEBUNKING LOBULAR CARCINOMA IN SITU

Although described by Foote and Stewart in 1941 as a "rare form of mammary cancer",[1] the entity they described was a intralobular lesion seen in association with invasive carcinoma **(Figure 5.1)**. "Pure" LCIS is typically an incidental finding with no clinical symptoms or signs. However, the introduction of national programs of breast-screening mammography has led to more frequent detection, and thus a seemingly increased incidence, of LCIS.[8] According to the surveillance, epidemiology and end results (SEER) database in the USA, by 2009 LCIS was being diagnosed in 2.75 per 100,000 women, aged 18–80.[6] Recent data from the Sloane Project suggests that in the UK screening population, the putative incidence of LN is 7 per 100,000, which is likely to be an underestimate.[8] The steady accumulation of data from these various cohorts is slowly challenging and or clarifying previous assumptions that were made about this disease. But, have we been able to comprehensively debunk LCIS?

Accepted wisdom is that LCIS is multifocal and bilateral

Since the 1970s, various studies have shown that a confirmed diagnosis of LCIS carries an equal risk (approximately 1% per year) of subsequent invasive breast cancer in either

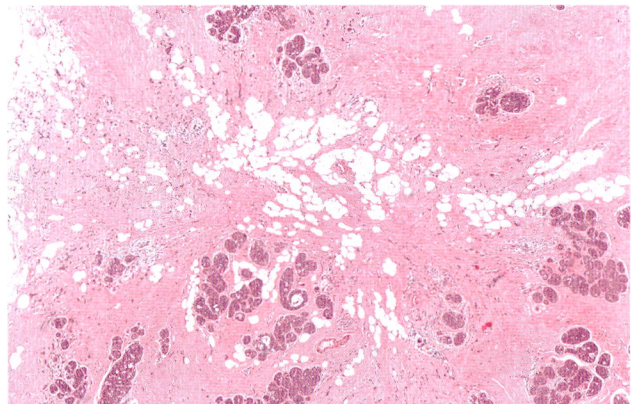

Figure 5.1 Hematoxylin and eosin-stained low-power view of breast excision with invasive lobular carcinoma of classical type and with adjacent lobular carcinoma in situ (LCIS).

breast.[4,6] Contralateral breast cancer may certainly occur in women with a previous diagnosis of LCIS, but the risk of developing an ipsilateral breast cancer is 2–3 times as high as that for contralateral disease.[4,9] Furthermore, LCIS is typically an incidental finding in benign breast biopsies (0.5–4%).[4,10,11] Thus, it is understandable, why the view that LCIS is multifocal in approximately one-third of cases and bilateral in another one-third has been perpetuated; contralateral breast cancer must arise because of an underestimation of the prevalence and extent of disease on imaging and core biopsy. But emerging evidence, although limited, suggests a somewhat different story.

In the Sloane Project report, which included 392 women with screen-detected pure LN accrued over a 10-year period, no cases of bilateral LN were registered.[8] Furthermore, King et al. reported an incidence of synchronous bilateral LCIS of only 2% in their longitudinal, surveillance study of women with LCIS presenting at Memorial Sloan-Kettering (MSK) between 1980 and 2009.[10] Indeed, of the 56 women who had bilateral prophylactic mastectomies, none were found to have bilateral LN.[10]

Houssami et al. investigated the accuracy and outcome of mammographic screening in women (n = 824) following a diagnosis of LN between 1996 and 2010.[12] Outcome data were collected either at 1-year postscreening or prior to the next screen (whichever came first) and were obtained from cancer registries and pathology reports. No central review was performed, unlike the series of King et al.[10] Nevertheless, 17 ipsilateral invasive cancers, 18 contralateral invasive cancers, and 2 bilateral breast cancers were reported.[12] In the same series, a population of women with a diagnosis of other forms of atypical hyperplasia (namely ductal, mixed, and "other") was also assessed (n = 1,743). In this latter cohort, 33 ipsilateral invasive cancers, 19 contralateral invasive cancers, and 7 bilateral breast cancers were found to have occurred within the same time frame.[12]

These data, albeit relatively limited, suggest that LN is not multifocal or bilateral as frequently as believed. Nevertheless, rarely, a genetic predisposition to bilateral LCIS exists; germline mutations in the E-cadherin gene, *CDH*1, have been shown to be associated with the early onset of bilateral LCIS, with or without invasive lobular carcinoma (ILC).[13]

Accepted wisdom is that all LCIS is equal

Variants of LCIS have been described, all of which characteristically show a loss of E-cadherin at a molecular level.[2,4,11] Of note, this is not necessarily reflected in complete absence of membranous E-cadherin positivity immunohistochemically, although this is often used by histopathologists in difficult cases to assess the disease. Of the types of LCIS identified, classical and pleomorphic LCIS are the two most common forms seen in routine diagnostic practice.[2-4,11,14,15]

In classical LCIS, the discohesive cells are typically moderately uniform, with small-to-moderately-sized nuclei[2,4,11] **(Figure 5.2)**. A moderate degree of nuclear atypia is typical (i.e. score "2" for atypia/pleomorphism). At a molecular level, classical LCIS is usually estrogen receptor (ER) positive, human epidermal growth factor receptor 2 (HER2) negative, lacks p53 mutation, and has a low-proliferation rate.[2,4]

The pleomorphic variant of LCIS (PLCIS) was first described in 1992.[16] This subtype is cytologically more reminiscent of high-grade ductal carcinoma in situ (DCIS); the nuclei are pleomorphic (i.e. score "3" for atypia/pleomorphism), the cells often have more abundant cytoplasm **(Figure 5.3)** and central, comedo-type necrosis may be present with associated microcalcification. Molecularly, despite showing the typically E-cadherin loss, PLCIS also shares features with DCIS. It can be ER negative, HER2 positive, show mutated p53, and can have an intermediate-to-high proliferation index.[2,4,11] An uncommon variant pleomorphic apocrine LCIS has also been described.

It seems logical, based on cytological and molecular features, that PLCIS may confer a greater risk of developing invasive malignancy than classical type LCIS. Unfortunately, this question remains somewhat unclear; no large-scale studies assessing the incidence and outcome of PLCIS have been performed. The finding that large numbers of isolated cases of "pure" PLCIS alone (i.e. with no concurrent invasive cancer) are difficult to collate supports the view that this lesion may progress relatively rapidly to invasive disease. In the largest three studies, comprising 32 cases of PLCIS in total, concurrent invasive cancer was present in 25–30% of patients.[11] It is undoubtedly the case that, prior to detailed pathological description and recognition of the entity, PLCIS would previously have been reported as high-grade DCIS and clinically managed as such.

At present, this approach, i.e. the same clinical management, of PLCIS to DCIS continues to be recommended.[11] Current Royal College of Pathologists and UK Breast Screening Program guidelines recommend that PLCIS, like DCIS, is classified as B5a when seen in core

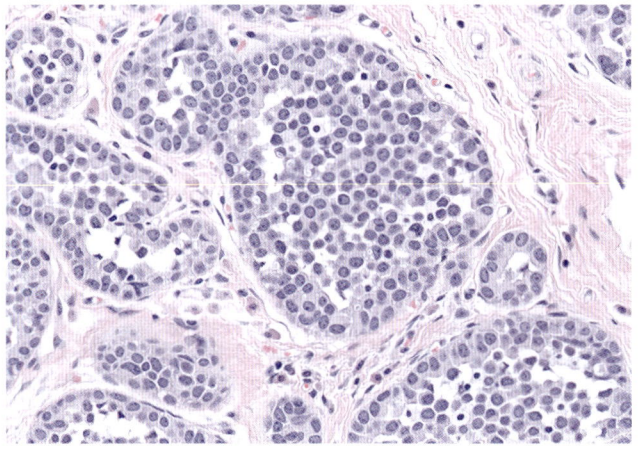

Figure 5.2 High-power hematoxylin and eosin-stained section of lobular carcinoma in situ (LCIS) of classical type. The moderately sized cells are discohesive (seen as clear spaces between the cells) but expand the space (more than eight cells across).

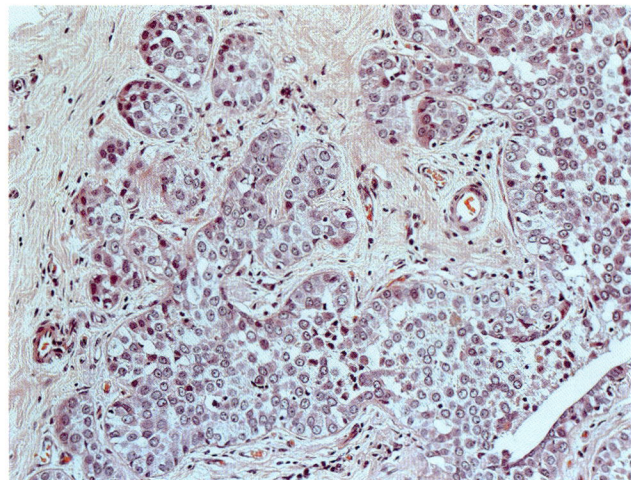

Figure 5.3 Pleomorphic lobular carcinoma in situ. The cells expanding the space are large and pleomorphic but have lobular, rather than ductal, cytological features including discohesion.

biopsy specimens. Typically, complete surgical excision is then recommended. There is, however, very little evidence regarding benefit of subsequent breast radiotherapy in patients undergoing breast-conserving therapy. Clinical trials assessing the management of PLCIS are required.

Other uncommon variants of LCIS, also with very limited clinical outcome data, have been described. One form shows admixed features of LCIS and DCIS (or both are unequivocally present) and cannot be accurately classified simply as either. This is not surprising, given the genetic similarities between these forms of in situ breast carcinoma and the increasingly recognized low-grade neoplasia family of lesions. Another form of classical LCIS with comedo-type necrosis has also been called florid LCIS or mass-forming LCIS and is seen histologically as cytologically classical LCIS (i.e. without marked pleomorphism) but with central comedo-type necrosis. For this reason, this type of disease may present mammographically with calcification. The most appropriate clinical management for both these variants (admixed DCIS and LCIS, and classical LCIS with necrosis) is not clear but both are presently managed as more akin to DCIS, based on the limited data available.

Accepted wisdom is that LCIS does not cause radiological abnormalities

Whether or not LCIS on its own causes a radiological abnormality has been the subject of much debate. Microcalcification has been consistently reported as the most common finding in association with both ALH and LCIS, being present in-between 60–70% of lesions biopsied.[9] In the Sloane Project series, the pattern of microcalcification was reported as usually punctate or granular in appearance (in >90% of the cases that had microcalcification); the type of calcification correlated with the size of the lesion; and a linear pattern was associated with larger lesions than granular or punctate patterns.[8] These series clearly only represent LN that has undergone biopsy and may not reflect the entire spectrum of disease.

A few studies have also recorded an association of LN with a mass or stromal deformity. The reason for this association is unclear and this may simply represent coexistence with another abnormality, at least in the majority. For this reason, Murray et al. suggested that the finding of LN in a core needle biopsy of a mammographic mass should be considered discordant.[17] However, there is some evidence that some LCIS may enhance on magnetic resonance imaging (MRI), and this, as well as the biology of the stroma surrounding such lesions, warrants further investigation.[18]

By comparing a population of patients with LN with matched controls, Houssami et al. calculated a mammographic screening sensitivity of 76.1% in the LN population, which did not significantly differ from the control cohort (82.3%; p = 0.43).[12] However, the specificity of mammography for LN (85.1%) was significantly lower than that of the control population (90.7%; p < 0.01). As noted, Murray et al. have suggested that discordance between radiology and pathology should be a cause for concern.[17] This approach will highlight potential sampling errors and those more likely to be upgraded at excision (e.g. a mass that is not explained by LN on core biopsy). In such cases repeat sampling, for example with vacuum-assisted technique, should be undertaken.

Accepted wisdom is that LCIS only increases the risk of malignancy, and is not a nonobligate precursor of invasive disease

It was previously believed that LCIS invariably gives rise to ILC. Data suggests that this is not correct; even though ILC is more common in women with a history of LCIS, the majority of cancers that develop in such women are invasive carcinomas of ductal/no special type (IDC).[2,4]

However, it has repeatedly been shown that both LCIS and ILC lose E-cadherin by either genetic (mutational loss) or epigenetic (methylation) mechanisms, resulting in the characteristic discohesion seen histologically.[2,19] There is a growing body of evidence supporting a shared clonal origin between LCIS and ILC, which over the years, has mirrored the increasing genomic resolution of ever-emerging technologies.[2,19,20] It is clear that LCIS shares a number of genetic aberrations with ILC, including whole arm chromosomal gains (at 1q) and losses (at 16q), and mutations, most frequently CDH1 and PIK3CA.

Begg et al. attempted tried to analyze whether LCIS shared a clonal origin with synchronous invasive carcinoma of ductal/no special type.[19] Unfortunately, the number of cases (n = 5) examined in the study was suboptimal, since most failed quality control for copy number analysis. However, using whole exome sequencing, they were able to demonstrate shared mutations in two of the cases. Interestingly, in one of the cases, the LCIS and IDC were in the same quadrant, while in the other, they were not. In the latter case, the woman also had an IDC that shared no mutations with LCIS in the same quadrant, but did with LCIS in a different quadrant. How to predict, which precursor lesions are more likely to progress to invasive malignancy is currently unknown.

What is even more fascinating is that, in this same study,[19] 15 women with multifocal and multicentric LCIS were also assessed to see if the various lesions were clonal; approximately two-thirds were clonal, while one-third were independent. Synchronous LCIS and DCIS from different quadrants of the breast were also analyzed, and most of these were also shown to be clonal. Since by definition, in situ lesions are contained by basement membrane and cannot move through the stroma, how is this possible? Does it point to the fact that any normal lobule or duct in the breast can only undergo a very limited number of genetic events in early carcinogenesis? Does it suggest that these changes may occur in parallel? Further studies are required to clarify these data and their significance. Nevertheless, it is generally now accepted that LCIS is a nonobligate precursor to invasive disease as well as an indicator of increased risk.

Accepted wisdom is that LCIS diagnosed on core biopsy requires surgical excision

Distinguishing LCIS from ALH is, as noted, based on extent and degree of the process in the terminal duct lobular units. As this cannot be undertaken with any reliability on the limited sampling inherent in core biopsy specimens, the recommendation in the UK is that the process is reported as LN and categorized as B3, of uncertain malignant potential. This is supported by the finding that the upgrade rate (i.e. the risk of any adjacent DCIS or invasive cancer contemporaneously) is essentially similar for cases categorized as ALH or as LCIS.[3] The upgrade rate in one UK based series was 29% following a diagnosis of LN on core biopsy[21] and in a larger meta-analysis was 27%.[3] For this reason, recent UK guidance is that further through sampling by vacuum-assisted technique is appropriate for all cases of LN diagnosed on needle core biopsy.[22] These recommend, if classical LN (B3) is diagnosed on small-bore needle core biopsy (i.e. 14 or 16 gauge) or vacuum-assisted biopsy, repeat vacuum-assisted excision/thorough sampling should be undertaken. In other words, the area of concern should be thoroughly sampled but surgical open biopsy is not required. These recommendations supersede the 2009 Association for Breast Surgery (ABS) guidelines that recommend that breast lesions containing LCIS "should be excised for definitive diagnosis as some patients may have a coexisting invasive malignancy".[23]

One study from the MD Anderson Cancer Center in 2014 proposed that management be directed by radiological–histological correlation.[9] Of 124 cases of classical LN, only 20 (16%) had surgical excision with an upgrade in 8 (40%). Significantly, however, the vast majority of the patients in this series had large-bore sampling (80% 9-gauge, 1% 10-gauge, and 8% 11-gauge) rather than 14- or 16-gauge small-bore needle sampling, with about two-thirds of women having 6–10 cores; in essence, an essentially similar approach to that now recommended in the UK.[22] They also, however, reported that a diagnostic upgrade was more common in lesions containing LCIS as opposed to ALH ($p = 0.002$), in extensive (involving ≥3 TDLUs) rather than focal lesions [although no focal lesions were excised ($p < 0.001$)] and in targeted rather than incidental lesions ($p < 0.001$). They also found that mass lesions rather than calcifications ($p = 0.011$) were more likely to be upgraded to DCIS or invasive carcinoma, supporting the view that multidisciplinary team discussion is essential in cases with a pathological diagnosis on core biopsy of LN (B3).

It is, however, certainly true that the generalizability of these studies addressing the upgrade rate of LN on core biopsy is limited.[3,24] Most studies looking at the rates of upgrade in women with LN provide only level III-2 evidence, and comprise studies with small sample sizes, that usually are retrospective and noncomparative in design. Many contain bias with regard to core biopsy needle sampling sizes and to ascertainment of patients (screening vs symptomatic) as well as variation in the proportion of women who have actually undergone surgical biopsy/excision of the lesion.

If there is no upgrade in the more extensively sampled tissue then surveillance as per a high-risk patient should continue, given the subsequent risk of development of carcinoma. The frequency and length and optimum modality of such surveillance is, however, less clear and requires research, although many centers advise annual mammography at present.

Accepted wisdom is that LCIS requires complete excision

The 2009 ABS guidelines[23] recommending that clear resection margins for classical LCIS are not required following surgery (since, it does not increase local recurrence) should be followed. Despite these national recommendations, in the Sloane Project analysis of LN, Maxwell et al. reported that the surgical procedures in 326 women with a final diagnosis of nonpleomorphic LN included 80 wide local excisions (3 with removal of the nipple), 3 mastectomies with two patients having up to 6 operations to clear margins.[8] These data clearly highlight that a subset of the screening population is being overtreated surgically at present. It is hoped, and expected, that these figures will change.

CONCLUSION

Although much progress has been made in recent years into understanding the biology and clinical course of LCIS, knowledge of precisely how one affects the other remains hindered by the relatively small number of studies performed and the relatively low incidence of this disease. It is to be hoped that new technologies (both for tissue sampling and for research) will allow for a more stratified approach to management women with LCIS.

> **Key points for clinical practice**
>
> - Classical LCIS, even when present at margins of excision, is not deemed to require complete surgical excision.
> - Evidence that LCIS is commonly multifocal and bilateral is not robust and subsequent ipsilateral breast cancer following a diagnosis of LCIS is two to three times more common than contralateral carcinoma.
> - PLCIS is regarded as a more aggressive form of LCIS, based on histological appearance and molecular profile, and more akin to high-grade DCIS.
> - Although there is limited evidence on clinical behavior, present management of PLCIS includes complete surgical excision.
> - Clinical trials to study optimum management of PLCIS are required.
> - While microcalcification may occasionally be associated with LCIS, multidisciplinary discussion is essential to identify cases of radiological–pathological discordance, which may indicate that the radiological abnormality has not been adequately sampled.
> - Lobular neoplasia (ALH or LCIS) identified on core biopsy is classified as B3 (unless pleomorphic variant, when it is categorized as B5a).
> - This diagnosis indicates a risk of adjacent associated DCIS or invasive carcinoma in the region of 20–30% and warrants further assessment.
> - Present guidelines recommend that this is by vacuum-assisted excision/thorough sampling rather than open surgical biopsy.
> - Research is required to assess the optimum mode, frequency, and length of follow-up surveillance for patients with a diagnosis of LCIS.

REFERENCES

1. Foote FW, Stewart FW. Lobular carcinoma in situ: A rare form of mammary cancer. Am J Pathol. 1941; 17(4):491-6.3.
2. O'Malley FP. Lobular neoplasia: morphology, biological potential and management in core biopsies. Mod Pathol. 2010;23(Suppl 2):S14-25.
3. Hussain M, Cunnick GH. Management of lobular carcinoma in-situ and atypical lobular hyperplasia of the breast—a review. Eur J Surg Oncol. 2011;37(4):279-89.
4. Morrow M, Schnitt SJ, Norton L. Current management of lesions associated with an increased risk of breast cancer. Nat Rev Clin Oncol. 2015;12(4):227-38.

5. McEvoy MP, Coopey SB, Mazzola E, et al. Breast cancer risk and follow-up recommendations for young women diagnosed with atypical hyperplasia and lobular carcinoma in situ (LCIS). Ann Surg Oncol. 2015;22(10):3346-9.
6. Portschy PR, Marmor S, Nzara R, et al. Trends in incidence and management of lobular carcinoma in situ: a population-based analysis. Ann Surg Oncol. 2013;20(10):3240-6.
7. Renshaw AA, Gould EW. Long term clinical follow-up of atypical ductal hyperplasia and lobular carcinoma in situ in breast core needle biopsies. Pathology. 2016;48(1):25-9.
8. Maxwell AJ, Clements K, Dodwell DJ, et al. The radiological features, diagnosis and management of screen-detected lobular neoplasia of the breast: Findings from the Sloane Project. Breast. 2016;27:109-15.
9. Middleton LP, Sneige N, Coyne R, et al. Most lobular carcinoma in situ and atypical lobular hyperplasia diagnosed on core needle biopsy can be managed clinically with radiologic follow-up in a multidisciplinary setting. Cancer Med. 2014;3(3):492-9.
10. King TA, Pilewskie M, Muhsen S, et al. Lobular carcinoma in situ: A 29-year longitudinal experience evaluating clinicopathologic features and breast cancer risk. J Clin Oncol. 2015;33(33):3945-52.
11. Carder PJ, Shaaban A, Alizadeh Y, et al. Screen-detected pleomorphic lobular carcinoma in situ (PLCIS): risk of concurrent invasive malignancy following a core biopsy diagnosis. Histopathology. 2010;57(3):472-8.
12. Houssami N, Abraham LA, Onega T, et al. Accuracy of screening mammography in women with a history of lobular carcinoma in situ or atypical hyperplasia of the breast. Breast Cancer Res Treat. 2014;145(3):765-73.
13. Petridis C, Shinomiya I, Kohut K, et al. Germline CDH1 mutations in bilateral lobular carcinoma in situ. Br J Cancer. 2014;110(4):1053-7.
14. Masannat YA, Bains SK, Pinder SE, et al. Challenges in the management of pleomorphic lobular carcinoma in situ of the breast. Breast. 2013;22(2):194-6.
15. Menon S, Porter GJ, Evans AJ, et al. The significance of lobular neoplasia on needle core biopsy of the breast. Virchows Arch. 2008;452(5):473-9.
16. Eusebi V, Magalhaes F, Azzopardi JG. Pleomorphic lobular carcinoma of the breast: an aggressive tumor showing apocrine differentiation. Hum Pathol. 1992;23(6):655-62.
17. Murray MP, Luedtke C, Liberman L, et al. Classic lobular carcinoma in situ and atypical lobular hyperplasia at percutaneous breast core biopsy: outcomes of prospective excision. Cancer. 2013;119(5):1073-9.
18. Schwartz T, Cyr A, Margenthaler J. Screening breast magnetic resonance imaging in women with atypia or lobular carcinoma in situ. J Surg Res. 2015;193(2):519-22.
19. Begg CB, Ostrovnaya I, Carniello JV, et al. Clonal relationships between lobular carcinoma in situ and other breast malignancies. Breast Cancer Res. 2016;18(1):66.
20. Logan GJ, Dabbs DJ, Lucas PC, et al. Molecular drivers of lobular carcinoma in situ. Breast Cancer Res. 2015;17:76.
21. Rakha EA, Lee AH, Jenkins JA, et al. Characterization and outcome of breast needle core biopsy diagnoses of lesions of uncertain malignant potential (B3) in abnormalities detected by mammographic screening. Int J Cancer. 2011;129(6):1417-24.
22. Public Health England. (2016). Appendix 2. Clinical guidance for breast cancer screening assessment. NHSBSP Publication 49, 4th edition. Public Health England. [online] Available from https://www.gov.uk/government/uploads/system/uploads/attachment_data/file/567600/Clinical_guidance_for_breast__cancer_screening__assessment_Nov_2016.pdf. [Accessed December, 2017].
23. Association of Breast Surgery at Baso 2009. Surgical guidelines for the management of breast cancer. Eur J Surg Oncol. 2009;35(Suppl 1):1-22.
24. Buckley ES, Webster F, Hiller JE, et al. A systematic review of surgical biopsy for LCIS found at core needle biopsy—do we have the answer yet? Eur J Surg Oncol. 2014;40(2):168-75.

Section 4

Head and Neck Surgery

CHAPTER

6. Neck Dissection in Head and Neck Cancers

Chapter 6

Neck dissection in head and neck cancers

Anshuman Singh, Akshay Anand, Abhinav Arun Sonkar

INTRODUCTION

Surgery has been the first-line management modality for most cancers of the head and neck except for cancers of a few primary sites such as posterior third of tongue, nasopharynx and a few subsites of the larynx. Chemotherapy and radiotherapy are used either as adjuncts to surgery or for palliation in cases of advanced disease, radiation has also been used as a modality equivalent to surgery in select cases. The surgical approach in any cancer of the head and neck involves resection of the primary tumor along with neck dissection for evaluation of the cervical lymph nodes for any evidence of metastasis, which if found involved, the expected survival is reduced to half. This highlights the significance of neck dissection as an equally important component of the treatment of any cancer of the head and neck. The extent of cervical lymph node dissection of cancers of the head and neck has long been a matter of debate. Their importance, evaluation strategies and recent developments are discussed under the subsequent sections.

IMPORTANCE OF LYMPHATIC INVOLVEMENT

Lymph node metastasis is the single most important prognostic factor in malignancies of the upper aerodigestive tract. More than 50% cases of squamous cell carcinoma of the oral cavity have lymph node metastases and the presence of nodal metastases reduces survival by nearly 50%.[1] Reports from the American Cancer Society indicate that squamous cell carcinomas (SCCs) of the oral cavity and pharynx have regionally disseminated disease in nearly 40% of patients.[2] Cancers of these regions are characterized by poor prognosis with an overall 5-year survival rate of only about 50–60% even after successful treatment of the primary tumor. This dismal outcome even after successful treatment of the primary tumor and poor long-term prognosis is probably due to high rates of regional recurrences due to inadequate treatment of lymphatic metastases which usually occur early in the course of the disease. The presence of regional lymph nodal metastases acts as an indicator of the ability of the primary tumor to metastasize locoregionally or systemically.[3] This may explain the dramatic fall in survival rate which occurs with the involvement of the locoregional lymph nodes in cancers of the head and neck. There is a continuous decrease in the 5-year survival rates as the stage of disease progresses from 83% in early stage (stage I and II), to 62% in regionally advanced disease (III, IVa, IVb) to approximately 38% in distant metastatic disease (stage IVc).[4] Early and regionally advanced disease can benefit from adequate dissection of the neck nodes with higher 5-year survival rates. Thus knowledge of locoregional lymphatic drainage and histopathological examination of cervical lymph nodes play the most important role in adequate control of disease alongside treatment of the primary tumor.

EVALUATION OF CERVICAL LYMPH NODES: DIAGNOSTIC DILEMMA IN CLINICALLY N0 (CN0) NECK

Lymphatic drainage of the head and neck involves a complex architecture of approximately 300 lymph nodes; as a result an assured diagnosis of lymphatic metastasis in primary tumors of the head and neck remains a challenge. Lymphatic metastasis from head and neck primaries usually occurs in a sequential and predictable manner. Patients with primary malignancy of the oral cavity with no clinical evidence of lymph nodal metastasis preoperatively are the patient group in which estimation of the pattern and sequence of nodal metastasis is required to decide on the extent of clearance of neck nodes required.

The risk of clinically undetectable micrometastasis in patients with clinically node-negative disease varies with different primary sites and so does the extent of lymph node clearance that is required. Furthermore, none of the current diagnostic modalities, including clinical examination, have adequate sensitivity and specificity to avoid the need for surgical staging of cervical lymph node status. The sensitivity of inspection and palpation alone for detection of cervical nodes is 60–70% while the corresponding values of magnetic resonance imaging (MRI) and computed tomography (CT) are between 65% and 88%.[5,6] Merritt et al.[7] in a systematic review of studies comparing palpation with CT found a sensitivity of 75% and 83% and a specificity of 81% and 83% for palpation and CT, respectively.

However, ultrasonography (US) allows a detailed evaluation of the intranodal architecture and when coupled with US guided aspiration cytology, its sensitivity and specificity are 80% and 98% respectively with the added advantage of repeatability whenever required.[8] Hence, US is considered superior to both CT and MRI for preoperative evaluation of lymphatic metastasis. However, 15–25% patients with occult micrometastasis in neck nodes could be missed even on sonography. Giancarlo et al.[9] comparing palpation with US found no difference between the methods with a sensitivity of only 82% and specificity of 80% for palpation. Haberal et al.[10] reported a sensitivity of 64%, 72%, and 81% and a specificity of 85%, 96% and 96%, for palpation, US and CT. The addition of positron emission tomography (PET) in the preoperative armamentarium has not been demonstrated to be superior to other modalities. A meta-analysis showed that PET examination may achieve a sensitivity of up to 80% and a specificity of 86%, although, it may miss nearly half of the cases which later prove to be positive for lymphatic metastasis, when neck dissection is performed.[11] The routine clinical application of PET for nodal evaluation of head and neck cancers including clinically N0 neck is not supported by the literature to date.[12] The only established advantage of PET-CT is in detection of residual disease post chemoradiation where it has a higher sensitivity and specificity than CT or MRI, with a higher negative predictive value for detection of malignancy. This has further been proven by retrospective pathological evaluation of neck dissection specimens post chemoradiation which demonstrated a correlation with PET scan results.[13,14] In patients who have a clinically negative neck post chemoradiation, PET-CT performed 12 weeks post chemotherapy is 90% reliable and further imaging becomes optional.[15,16] For patients with equivocal PET-CT results, a recent study suggests a repeat PET-CT 4–6 weeks later may help to identify those patients who can be safely kept under observation without the need for surgery for suspected disease progression or residual disease.[17]

The gold standard for evaluation of neck nodes is histopathological examination after neck dissection. The 15–25% of patients that harbor occult micrometastases (<2 mm) may be missed on routine microscopic examination. Immunohistochemistry for cytokeratin 5 and 14, are an important adjunct to the routine microscopic examination in the detection of such cases. Another option is the use of quantitative RT-PCR for cytokeratins in nodal specimens. Although it may further improve the diagnostic accuracy for the occult micrometastasis[18,19] its routine use has been questioned keeping in mind the cost-effectiveness of the procedure.

EVOLUTION OF SURGERY FOR CERVICAL LYMPH NODE METASTASES

Neck dissection, as first described by Jawdynski in the 19th century underwent several changes until Crile described the concept of "radical neck dissection" (RND) in 1905 and this has been the gold standard for clinically palpable neck metastasis for many decades. It involves removal of ipsilateral levels I to V nodes along with the sternocleidomastoid muscle, internal jugular vein, and spinal accessory nerve (SAN). This procedure though oncologically superior was associated with significant postoperative morbidity. Most distressing was the classical "shoulder syndrome" due to sacrifice of the SAN which resulted in shoulder droop, scapular dyskinesia and pain around the shoulder joint. In 1962, Suarez introduced the concept of modified radical neck dissection (MRND); with preservation of sternocleidomastoid, internal jugular vein and the SAN, either one, two or all of these structures. The biggest advantage of MRND was preservation of SAN. The change in surgical technique is intrinsic to the philosophy of preventive treatment and led to dramatic improvement in the postoperative functional and cosmetic results without significant loss in the therapeutic efficacy. The advent of MRND led to sparing of the SAN, which due to the prevention of shoulder syndrome led to a considerable reduction in postoperative morbidity associated with RND without any significant reduction in the therapeutic efficacy. Subsequently, an improved understanding of the pattern of lymphatic spread in neck nodes led to conservation of uninvolved nodes, a concept that was called selective neck dissection. It involved removal of only those levels, which were at highest risk of metastasis while sparing the rest of the nodes unlike RND and MRND, which involved removal of all nodes from level, I to V irrespective of their involvement. As of now, surgery for cervical nodal metastases can be broadly classified into two categories for better understanding: (1) comprehensive neck dissection (for clinically N+ cases) and (2) selective neck dissection (for clinically N0 cases).[20]

Comprehensive neck dissection involves the surgical removal of all the structures in the lateral aspect of neck and includes the following procedures:
- Classic RND (levels I to V nodes, sternocleidomastoid muscle, internal jugular vein, SAN, and submandibular salivary gland)
- Extended RND (i.e. resection of additional regional lymph nodes or sacrifice of other structures such as cranial nerves, muscles, or skin in addition to the structures removed in classical RND)
- Modified radical neck dissection type I (MRND-I), with selective preservation of the SAN
- Modified radical neck dissection type II (MRND-II), with preservation of the SAN and the sternocleidomastoid muscle but resection of the internal jugular vein.
- Modified radical neck dissection type III (MRND-III), with preservation of the SAN, internal jugular vein, and sternocleidomastoid muscle.

Selective neck dissection involves removal of selected groups of lymph nodes at risk of micrometastasis in a clinically N0 neck.[21,22] This operation comprises:
- Supraomohyoid neck dissection (SOHND), which encompasses dissection of lymph nodes at levels I, II, and III (and sometimes superior portion of level IV)[20] preferred in SCCs of oral cavity.

- Jugular node dissection, which includes dissection of lymph nodes at levels II, III, and IV preferred in primary tumors of pharynx.
- Anterolateral neck dissection, which includes dissection of lymph nodes at levels I, II, III, and IV preferred in primary tumors of tongue.
- Posterolateral neck dissection, which includes lymph nodes in the suboccipital triangle, posterior triangle of the neck, level V, and the deep jugular chain of lymph nodes at levels II, III, and IV for melanomas and squamous carcinomas of the posterior scalp.
- Central compartment neck dissection, which involves clearance of lymph nodes at level VI in the central compartment of the neck adjacent to the thyroid gland and in the tracheoesophageal groove for thyroid cancer preferred in thyroid malignancies.

THERAPEUTIC APPROACH IN CLINICALLY N0 CANCERS: ROLE OF ELECTIVE VERSUS THERAPEUTIC NECK DISSECTION

The question arises as to why in clinically N0 neck, the nodes need to be treated? When lymph node involvement is not found clinically or by imaging, but the risk of microscopic metastases (15–20% or more) is higher than the risk associated with addition of a surgical procedure and its morbidity, neck dissection becomes a viable option.

The involvement of lymph nodes is dependent on many factors which includes the T stage which reflects tumor burden or invasiveness and is thus correlated with the risk of nodal metastasis for any given primary site.[3] Overall, the risk for metastasis is less than 15% for T1, 15–30% for T2, 30–50% for T3 and up to 75% for T4 head and neck primary SCCs. For a particular T stage, the subset of disease with endophytic and poorly differentiated tumors have greater risk of nodal metastasis than exophytic and well-differentiated tumors respectively **(Flowchart 6.1)**. Tumor thickness, however, is considered an independent risk factor for nodal metastasis in tumors of tongue and floor of mouth with 4 mm being considered the cut off, with thicker tumors bearing greater risk.[3]

Diagnostically the most definite approach for accurate evaluation of cervical lymph nodes is histopathological examination of the lymph nodes. The timing of neck dissection in clinically N0 neck has been a matter of debate for a long time. Whether to perform prophylactic "elective" neck dissection at the time of primary surgery or following a close wait and watch policy after excision of the primary tumor and performing "therapeutic" neck dissection only once nodal relapse occurs, has been a long-standing debate. Both procedures have their merits and drawbacks. Elective dissection has many advantages such as accurate evaluation of occult micrometastases, delineation of the extent of lymphatic metastases and identification of poor prognostic factors for nodal recurrence (extracapsular spread, perineural or perivascular invasion, tumor emboli in lymphatics, central necrosis) and consequently selecting the patients for adjuvant radiotherapy. On the other hand, it leads to high number of negative neck dissections and associated morbidity. Therapeutic neck dissection has the advantage of avoiding unnecessary neck dissections but with the associated risk of nodal relapse, which may sometimes be advanced enough to be inoperable.

Studies to date do not provide a definitive indication to support management decision-making. The most effective way to evaluate the usefulness of elective neck dissection is to conduct a randomized controlled trial (RCT). To date there are 5 RCTs performed with this objective. Vandenbrouck et al.[23] in a randomized setting showed no significant advantage of elective neck dissection over close observation and follow-up. Fakih et al.[24] in their study

Flowchart 6.1 Algorithm for management of neck nodes in primary squamous cell carcinomas (SCCs) of head and neck.

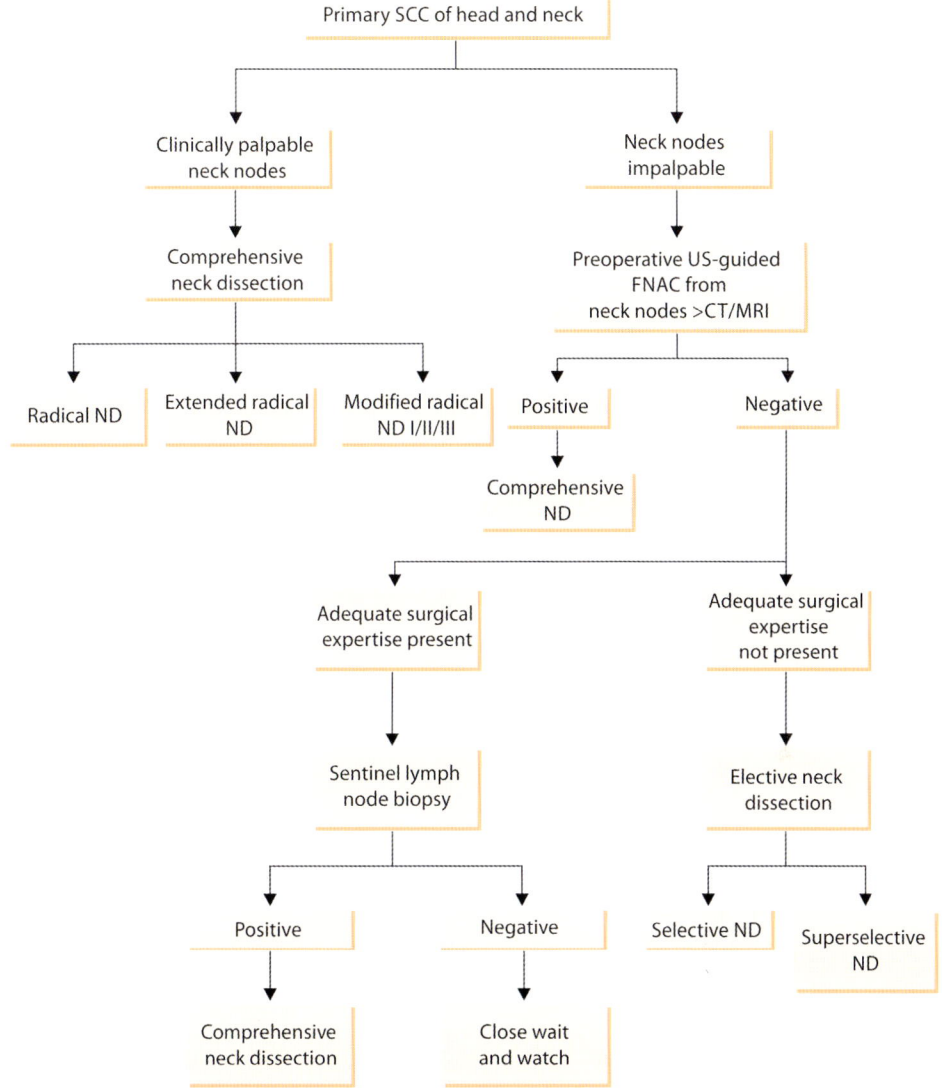

(FNAC: Fine-needle aspiration cytology; CT: Computed tomography; MRI: Magnetic resonance imaging; ND: Neck dissection).

indicated therapeutic advantage in terms of better overall and disease-free survival for the group of elective neck dissection. Kligerman et al.[25] in another randomized study with 67 cases and recently a multicenter randomized trial by Yuen et al.[26] described similar results in favor of elective neck dissection. The results in all the above-mentioned studies had limitations of small sample size. In 2015, D'Cruz et al.[27] in a large randomized study brought an end to the controversy when their analysis of 496 patients clearly proved an absolute overall survival benefit of 12.5% and a disease-free survival benefit of 23.6% for elective neck dissection in clinically N0 SCCs of the oral cavity over close wait and watch policy followed by therapeutic neck dissection at the time of nodal relapse. The superior benefit in the trial led to early termination of the study. Recently a meta-analysis combining the above five RCTs concluded there was an overall as well as disease-free survival benefit in favor of elective neck dissection.[28] Thus the evidence to date favors elective neck dissection performed at the time of resection of the primary tumor, which confers an overall survival benefit in patients with early stage, clinically node-negative oral squamous cell carcinoma. The extent of elective neck dissection to be carried out depends on the associated risk of lymphatic metastasis, which in turn depends on the location, and extent of the primary tumor as previously discussed. In primary tumors of the oral cavity with cN0 neck, the highest chance of nodal metastases is to the levels I to III lymph node levels and it is very rare for skip metastasis to occur to levels IV or V in the absence of involvement of level I, II or III. The incidence of skip metastases at level IV rises from 3% to 28%, depending upon the specific site of the primary tumor.[29,30]

As a result, in a clinically node-negative disease with primary tumor of the oral cavity, selective clearance of the levels I, II and III (supraomohyoid neck dissection) is usually sufficient without the need for comprehensive neck dissection. For cancers of the body of the tongue dissection should also involve removal of level IV lymph nodes keeping in mind the greater metastatic potential and more aggressive nature of the disease probably due to greater density of lymphatics. Studies have even reported isolated involvement of level IV lymph nodes only (skip metastasis) in primary lesions of the tongue in 10% of cases without involvement of level I to III lymph nodes. Similarly for primary tumors of the lateral part of oropharynx, hypopharynx and larynx with clinically undetectable nodes, the highest chances for micrometastasis is to the levels II, III, and IV with rare chance of skip metastasis to level I or V. Involvement of level V with primary lesions of oral cavity and clinically negative nodes is exceedingly rare. Thus in cases of clinically N0 of head and neck cancer, selective neck dissection is performed and it has been proven in many studies that nodal metastasis beyond the confines of an appropriate selective neck dissection is rare (<10%).[30-32]

LEVEL IIB DISSECTION AND ROLE OF SUPER SELECTIVE NECK DISSECTION

Level IIB removal has generated a lot of controversy and is discussed in the literature bearing in mind the high-risk of injury to the SAN during dissection of this group, as well as the low probability of its involvement in lymphatic metastasis of head and neck primaries. In selective neck dissection, shoulder function impairment has been observed in 21–60% of cases despite preservation of the SAN.[33,34] This functional injury despite anatomic integrity is probably due to close proximity of the SAN to the level IIB nodes and stretching of the nerve due to dissection performed in its vicinity. Level IIB nodal metastasis has been documented to be 5–10% in cN0 neck undergoing elective neck dissection.[35-37] It has also been stated that the oral cavity does not drain directly into level IIB[20,38,39] and also it is rarely involved in isolation. When involved it is accompanied by either clinically identifiable metastasis to other levels or occult metastasis of level IIA.

In a recent study, de Vicente et al.[40] described the prevalence of metastasis at level IIB was 0% in pathological proven N0 necks and 3.4% in pathological N+ necks, with an overall prevalence of 1.8% in oral cancer. Villaret et al.[41] in a multicentric trial has stated that the oral cavity has the highest overall prevalence of level IIB metastasis (10%) among head and neck SCCs, but these metastases are only found in 2% of cN0 cases. Pantvaidya et al.[42]

described similar findings in tongue cancers (5%) and cancers of the retromolar trigone (6.2%) as subsites. Based on a meta-analysis, the frequency of nodal metastasis to level IIB in previously untreated OSCC is 6.0% (95% CI: 3.5–8.6).[43] Based on these findings, it can be concluded that inclusion of level IIB when performing elective neck dissection in cN0 cases might be unnecessary and can be avoided without significant risk of relapse, to prevent postoperative shoulder disability.

It has been established that an appropriately indicated selective neck dissection can achieve the same oncologic outcomes as modified therapeutic ones. An even more explicit neck dissection, termed superselective neck dissection, involves the compartmental removal of the fibrofatty tissue contents within the defined boundaries of two or fewer contiguous neck levels. Evidence from retrospective studies suggests that superselective neck dissection is oncologically proposed for two indications: (1) elective treatment of clinically N0 neck and (2) salvage treatment of persistent lymph node disease after chemoradiotherapy.[44] Evidence-based trials with a large number of cases can justify the idea of this type of neck dissection, which is presently a futuristic concept. This concept has led to further investigation of the role of preserving level IIB nodes during selective neck dissection for oral cavity cancers (other than cancer tongue) with clinically N0 neck to prevent SAN related injury. Robbins et al. have indicated that selective and superselective neck dissection, which spare function and minimize morbidity, are viable therapeutic alternatives for patients with residual disease confined to 1 level after various chemoradiation protocols.[45]

ROLE OF SENTINEL LYMPH NODE SAMPLING

The significance of sentinel node sampling was brought into consideration with the aim to reduce the need for elective neck dissection to a minimum, so as to prevent the morbidities associated with it. In head and neck cancers the complex lymphatic architecture and the high density of lymph nodes in the region resulted in failure to accurately determine the first draining nodes. As a result, some authors were of the opinion to remove at least 2–3 sentinel lymph nodes in order to exclude the false-negative results.[19] In an evaluation performed at the Department of Otolaryngology, Marburg, Germany, sampling of only one sentinel lymph node was associated with a false-negative rate of nearly 40%.[46] These results when compared with the complexity of dissection required in the sampling of sentinel nodes often in rather inaccessible areas and subsequent risks of intraoperative damage to non-lymphatic structures, do not support the use of sentinel node biopsy for evaluation of neck nodes in clinically N0 cancers in centers where surgical expertise is inadequate. Thus, as of now, selective node dissection at the time of primary surgery (elective neck dissection) seems to be a better alternative for a staging procedure rather than sentinel lymph node biopsy in centers where surgical expertise for sentinel node biopsy is not available. In centers with adequate surgical expertise, sentinel lymph node biopsy may be considered prior to neck dissection for histopathological examination in cases of cN0 head and neck cancers.

NATIONAL COMPREHENSIVE CANCER NETWORK 2016 GUIDELINES FOR HEAD AND NECK CANCERS

In the 7th edition of the American Joint Committee on Cancer (AJCC) staging manual, the words *resectable* and *unresectable* with respect to head and neck malignancies have been replaced by the terms moderately advanced, i.e. T4a and *very advanced*, i.e. T4b.[47] The reason is that there has never been a consensus regarding the *resectability* of any given tumor and it depends to a reasonable extent on the surgical expertise available and existing medical comorbidities. Thus, a designation of stage IV does not always designate unresectable disease. The National Comprehensive Cancer Network (NCCN) panel, in general, recommends single modality treatment with either surgery or radiotherapy for early stage cancers (stage I and II) and combined modality therapy for locally or regionally advanced disease (stage III and IV). However the final decision is guided by the specific site of the primary, stage and the pathologic findings. For neck dissection, NCCN follows the contemporary nomenclature of comprehensive and selective neck dissection based on the number of lymph node groups that are resected.[21] As per the NCCN guidelines, the chief role of selective neck dissections is to determine the patients who are candidates for possible adjuvant therapy (CT/RT or RT alone), although it may be used as treatment when the tumor burden is low, i.e. clinically N0,[48] whilst in cases with neck node metastasis comprehensive neck dissection is the preferred surgical modality. Sentinel node biopsy, although less accurate for floor of mouth cancers,[49,50] can help to identify occult cervical metastases[51-54] and can avoid the morbidities associated with neck dissection in cN0 neck and should be performed in centers with adequate surgical expertise.

CONCLUSION

The extent of lymph node metastasis is the single most important prognostic factor for head and neck cancer. US guided FNAC has been shown to be superior to CT and MRI but histopathological examination of neck nodes still remains the gold standard for assessment of nodal metastasis. The extent of neck dissection depends on the risk of lymphatic metastasis, i.e. site, extent and histomorphology of the primary tumor. Comprehensive and selective neck dissections should be performed when indicated. Elective node dissection has improved efficacy in terms of survival in clinically negative necks. Specific indications for sentinel lymph node biopsy and superselective dissection are still under evaluation.

> **Key points for clinical practice**
>
> - Extent of lymph node metastasis is the most important prognostic factor for head and neck SCC.
> - US guided fine-needle aspiration cytology (FNAC) from neck nodes is superior to both CT and MRI scans for detection of nodal metastasis.
> - Histopathological examination of neck nodes is gold standard for assessment of nodal metastasis.
> - Immunohistochemistry is useful adjunct to HPE for detection of micrometastasis.
> - Comprehensive neck dissection is indicated in clinically palpable cervical lymph nodes.
> - Selective neck dissection is indicated in clinically undetectable cervical lymph nodes.
> - Elective neck dissection is superior to therapeutic neck dissection in cN0 SCC of the oral cavity.
> - The extent of neck dissection depends on the risk of lymphatic metastasis, i.e. site, extent and histomorphology of the primary tumor, i.e. elective neck dissection is selective neck dissection.
> - Level IIB lymph nodes could be safely excluded while performing elective neck dissection in cN0 SCC of the oral cavity without significant risk of relapse.
> - Sentinel LN biopsy could be used in place of elective neck dissection for diagnostic evaluation of neck nodes provided adequate surgical expertise is available.

REFERENCES

1. Shah JP, Patel SG, Singh B. Cervical lymph nodes. In: Shah JP, Patel SG, Singh B (Eds). Jatin Shah's Head and Neck Surgery and Oncology, 4th edition. Philadelphia: Elsevier; 2012. p. 426.
2. American Cancer Society. Cancer Facts and Figures 2016. Atlanta: American Cancer Society; 2016.
3. Paleri V, Watkinson JC. Metastatic neck disease. In: Watkinson JC, Gilbert RW (Eds). Stell and Maran's Textbook of Head and Neck Surgery and Oncology, 5th edition. UK: Hodder Arnold; 2012. p. 663.
4. National Cancer Institute. (2016). SEER Cancer Statistics Review, 1975-2013. [online] Available from https://seer.cancer.gov/archive/csr/1975_2013.
5. van den Brekel MW, Castelijns JA, Stel HV, et al. Modern imaging techniques and ultrasound-guided aspiration cytology for the assessment of neck node metastases: a prospective comparative study. Eur Arch Otorhinolaryngol. 1993;250:11-7.
6. de Bondt RB, Nelemans PJ, Hofman PA, et al. Detection of lymph node metastases in head and neck cancer: a meta-analysis comparing US, USgFNAC, CT and MR imaging. Eur J Radiol. 2007;64:266-72.
7. Merritt RM, Williams MF, James TH, et al. Detection of cervical metastasis. A meta-analysis comparing computed tomography with physical examination. Arch Otolaryngol Head Neck Surg. 1997;123:149-52.
8. Kyzas PA, Evangelou E, Denaxa-Kyza D, et al. 18F-fluorodeoxyglucose positron emission tomography to evaluate cervical node metastases in patients with head and neck squamous cell carcinoma: a meta-analysis. J Natl Cancer Inst. 2008;100:712-20.
9. Giancarlo T, Palmieri A, Giacomarra V, et al. Preoperative evaluation of cervical adenopathies in tumours of the upper aerodigestive tract. Anticancer Res. 1998;18:2805-9.
10. Haberal I, Celik H, Gocmen H, et al. Which is important in the evaluation of metastatic lymph nodes in head and neck cancer: palpation, ultrasonography, or computed tomography? Otolaryngol Head Neck Surg. 2004;130:197-201.
11. Yao M, Graham MM, Hoffman HT, et al. The role of post-radiation therapy FDG PET in prediction of necessity for post-radiation therapy neck dissection in locally advanced head- and-neck squamous cell carcinoma. Int J Radiat Oncol Biol Phys. 2004;59:1001-10.
12. Nahmias C, Carlson ER, Duncan LD, et al. Positron emission tomography/computerized tomography (PET/CT) scanning for preoperative staging of patients with oral/head and neck cancer. J Oral Maxillofac Surg. 2007;65:2524-35.
13. Ong SC, Schöder H, Lee NY, et al. Clinical utility of 18F-FDG PET/CT in assessing the neck after concurrent chemoradiotherapy for Locoregional advanced head and neck cancer. J Nucl Med. 2008;49:532-40.
14. Rinaldo A, Devaney KO, Ferlito A. Immunohistochemical studies in the identification of lymph node micrometastases in patients with squamous cell carcinoma of the head and neck. ORL J Otorhinolaryngol Relat Spec. 2004;66:38-41.
15. Nayak JV, Walvekar RR, Andrade RS, et al. Deferring planned neck dissection following chemoradiation for stage IV head and neck cancer: the utility of PET-CT. Laryngoscope. 2007;117:2129-34.
16. Abgral R, Querellou S, Potard G, et al. Does 18F-FDG PET/CT improve the detection of posttreatment recurrence of head and neck squamous cell carcinoma in patients negative for disease on clinical follow-up? J Nucl Med. 2009;50:24-9.
17. Porceddu SV, Pryor DI, Burmeister E, et al. Results of a prospective study of positron emission tomography-directed management of residual nodal abnormalities in node-positive head and neck cancer after definitive radiotherapy with or without systemic therapy. Head Neck. 2011;33:1675-82.
18. Becker MT, Shores CG, Yu KK, et al. Molecular assay to detect metastatic head and neck squamous cell carcinoma. Arch Otolaryngol Head Neck Surg. 2004;130:21-7.
19. Werner JA, Dünne AA, Brandt D, et al. [Studies on significance of sentinel lymphadenectomy in pharyngeal and laryngeal carcinoma]. Laryngorhinootologie. 1999;78:663-70.
20. Robbins KT, Shaha AR, Medina JE, et al. Consensus statement on the classification and terminology of neck dissection. Arch Otolaryngol Head Neck Surg. 2008;134:536-8.
21. Byers RM. Neck dissection: concepts, controversies, and technique. Semin Surg Oncol. 1991;7:9-13.
22. Stringer SP. Current concepts in surgical management of neck metastases from head and neck cancer. Oncology (Williston Park). 1995;9:547-54.
23. Vandenbrouck C, Sancho-garnier H, Chassagne D, et al. Elective versus therapeutic radical neck dissection in epidermoid carcinoma of the oral cavity: results of a randomized clinical trial. Cancer. 1980;46:386-90.

24. Fakih AR, Rao RS, Borges AM, et al. Elective versus therapeutic neck dissection in early carcinoma of the oral tongue. Am J Surg. 1989;158:309-13.
25. Kligerman J, Lima RA, Soares JR, et al. Supraomohyoid neck dissection in the treatment of T1/T2 squamous cell carcinoma of oral cavity. Am J Surg. 1994;168:391-4.
26. Yuen AP, Ho CM, Chow TL, et al. Prospective randomized study of selective neck dissection versus observation for N0 neck of early tongue carcinoma. Head Neck. 2009;31:765-72.
27. D'Cruz AK, Vaish R, Kapre N, et al. Elective versus therapeutic neck dissection in node-negative oral cancer. New Engl J Med. 2015;373:521-9.
28. Zhen-Hu Ren, Jian-Lin Xu, Bo Li, et al. Elective versus therapeutic neck dissection in node-negative oral cancer: Evidence from five randomized controlled trials. Oral Oncol. 2015;51:976-81.
29. Byers RM, Weber RS, Andrews T, et al. Frequency and therapeutic implications of "skip metastases" in the neck from squamous carcinoma of the oral tongue. Head Neck. 1997;19:14-9.
30. Shah JP, Candela FC, Poddar AK. The patterns of cervical lymph node metastases from squamous carcinoma of the oral cavity. Cancer. 1990;66:109-13.
31. Candela FC, Kothari K, Shah JP. Patterns of cervical node metastases from squamous carcinoma of the oropharynx and hypopharynx. Head Neck. 1990;12:197-203.
32. Candela FC, Shah J, Jaques DP, et al. Patterns of cervical node metastases from squamous carcinoma of the larynx. Arch Otolaryngol Head Neck Surg. 1990;116:432-5.
33. Short SO, Kaplan JN, Laramore GE, et al. Shoulder pain and function after neck dissection with or without preservation of the spinal accessory nerve. Am J Surg. 1984;148:478-82.
34. Talmi YP, Hoffman HT, Horowitz Z, et al. Patterns of metastases to the upper jugular lymph nodes (the "submuscular recess"). Head Neck. 1998;20:682-6.
35. Lim YC, Song MH, Kim SC, et al. Preserving level IIb lymph nodes in elective supraomohyoid neck dissection for oral cavity squamous cell carcinoma. Arch Otolaryngol Head Neck Surg. 2004;130:1088-91.
36. Elsheikh MN, Mahfouz ME, Elsheikh E. Level IIB lymph nodes metastasis in elective supraomohyoid neck dissection for oral cavity squamous cell carcinoma: a molecular-based study. Laryngoscope. 2005;115:1636-40.
37. Cheng PT, Hao SP, Lin YH, et al. Objective comparison of shoulder dysfunction after three neck dissection techniques. Ann Otol Rhinol Laryngol. 2000;109:761-6.
38. Shah JP. Patterns of cervical lymph node metastasis from squamous carcinomas of the upper aerodigestive tract. Am J Surg. 1990;160:405-9.
39. Woolgar JA. Histological distribution of cervical lymph node metastases from intraoral/oropharyngeal squamous cell carcinomas. Br J Oral Maxillofac Surg. 1999;37:175-80.
40. de Vicente JC, Rodríguez-Santamarta T, Peña I, et al. Relevance of level IIB neck dissection in oral squamous cell carcinoma. Med Oral Patol Oral Cir Bucal. 2015;20:e547-53.
41. Villaret AB, Piazza C, Peretti G, et al. Multicentric prospective study on the prevalence of sublevel IIB metastases in head and neck cancer. Arch Otolaryngol Head Neck Surg. 2007;133:897-903.
42. Pantvaidya GH, Pal P, Vaidya AD, et al. Prospective study of 583 neck dissections in oral cancers: implications for clinical practice. Head Neck. 2014;36:1503-7.
43. Lea J, Bachar G, Sawka AM, et al. Metastases to level IIB in squamous cell carcinoma of the oral cavity: a systematic review and meta-analysis. Head Neck. 2010;32:184-90.
44. Suárez C, Rodrigo JP, Robbins KT, et al. Superselective neck dissection: rationale, indications, and results. Eur Arch Otorhinolaryngol. 2013;270:2815-21.
45. Robbins KT, Doweck I, Samant S, et al. Effectiveness of superselective and selective neck dissection for advanced nodal metastases after chemoradiation. Arch Otolaryngol Head Neck Surg. 2005;131:965-9.
46. Werner JA, Dünne AA, Ramaswamy A, et al. The sentinel node concept in head and neck cancer: solution for the controversies in the N0 neck? Head Neck. 2004;26:603-11.
47. Edge S, Byrd D, Compton C, et al. AJCC Cancer Staging Manual, 7th edition. New York: Springer; 2010.
48. Ferlito A, Rinaldo A, Silver CE, et al. Elective and therapeutic selective neck dissection. Oral Oncol. 2006;42:14-25.
49. Alkureishi LW, Ross GL, Shoaib T, et al. Sentinel node biopsy in head and neck squamous cell cancer: 5-year follow-up of a European multicenter trial. Ann Surg Oncol. 2010;17:2459-64.
50. Civantos FJ, Zitsch RP, Schuller DE, et al. Sentinel lymph node biopsy accurately stages the regional lymph nodes for T1-T2 oral squamous cell carcinomas: results of a prospective multi-institutional trial. J Clin Oncol. 2010;28:1395-400.

51. Govers TM, Hannink G, Merkx MA, et al. Sentinel node biopsy for squamous cell carcinoma of the oral cavity and oropharynx: a diagnostic meta-analysis. Oral Oncol. 2013;49:726-32.
52. Samant S. Sentinel node biopsy as an alternative to elective neck dissection for staging of early oral carcinoma. Head Neck. 2014;36:241-6.
53. Broglie MA, Haerle SK, Huber GF, et al. Occult metastases detected by sentinel node biopsy in patients with early oral and oropharyngeal squamous cell carcinomas: impact on survival. Head Neck. 2013;35:660-6.
54. Pezier T, Nixon IJ, Gurney B, et al. Sentinel lymph node biopsy for T1/T2 oral cavity squamous cell carcinoma—a prospective case series. Ann Surg Oncol. 2012;19:3528-33.

Section 5

Upper Gastrointestinal Surgery

CHAPTER

7. Penetrating Trauma of the Upper Gastrointestinal Tract: Practical Notes on Surgical Management

Chapter 7

Penetrating trauma of the upper gastrointestinal tract: Practical notes on surgical management

Frank Plani

INTRODUCTION

The upper gastrointestinal tract (GIT) comprises the buccal cavity, pharynx, esophagus, stomach and duodenum—separation from the lower intestinal tract being provided by the ligament of Treitz. Its structures are therefore part of the face, neck, chest, and abdominal cavity, including the retroperitoneum. Most injuries of the mouth and pharynx will be managed by ear, nose, and throat (ENT) or maxillofacial specialists and will not be considered in this chapter. General surgical trainees and consultants not actively involved in trauma are the least comfortable with operating in the neck and the thorax, and therefore most of this chapter will focus on these regions.[1]

ANATOMICAL NOTES

Neck

The surgical approach to the neck in penetrating trauma is often a race against time in the presence of exsanguinating bleeding or expanding hematomas. For many surgeons, this is unfamiliar, unforgiving territory due to the close proximity of neurovascular and aerodigestive structures. Furthermore, all these structures lie within the two layers of cervical fascia, deep and superficial, which places the airway at risk from hematomas.

Bleeding into the airways or collapse and obliteration of the airways can occur unexpectedly upon initiation of intubation, and preparation for a difficult airway and requirement for a surgical airway must always be made. The concept of surgical airway in neck trauma frequently goes beyond cricothyrotomy and may require an emergency low tracheostomy.[2]

In order to give guidance on how to approach nonspinal neck injuries, the neck (anterior to the sternomastoid muscle) can be divided into three zones, based on the ease of proximal and distal vascular control. As far as the aerodigestive structures are concerned:
1. *Zone 1* extends between the clavicle and the cricoid cartilage, containing the origin of the esophagus and the trachea.
2. *Zone II* is between the cricoid cartilage and the angle of the mandible.
3. *Zone III* goes up to the skull base, comprising both the pharynx and the larynx.

Table 7.1: American Association for the Surgery of Trauma (AAST) Organ Injury Scale–Lacerations–Esophagus.	
Grade 1	Partial thickness, not into lumen, and serosal tear
Grade 2	Laceration into lumen, <50% of diameter
Grade 3	Laceration of >50% of the diameter
Grade 4	Segmental loss or devascularization <2 cm
Grade 5	Segmental loss or devascularization >2 cm

The use of zones, while very relevant in the pre-computerized tomography (CT) scan era, has lost a lot of its clinical meaning when utilizing CT scans extensively before any surgery.[3,4] However, in the unstable patient who cannot go to the CT scanner, it is still very relevant, since it indicates the necessity to perform a sternotomy for proximal control in a Zone 1 injury, and prepare for a difficult exposure of the base of the skull, up to the mastoid, for distal control in a Zone 3 injury.[5,6]

Chest and abdomen

The esophagus travels from slightly to the left of the midline in the neck to enter the right chest cavity and lie to the right of the descending aorta, underneath the azygos vein, abutting the membranous trachea and the posterior pericardium further down. The recurrent laryngeal nerves travel in the tracheoesophageal grooves. The esophagus then enters the diaphragm through the esophageal hiatus at the level of T10 or T11.

The American Association for the Surgery of Trauma (AAST) Organ Injury Scale—Lacerations can be adapted for the esophagus with one extra grade for multiple injuries up to Grade 3 **(Table 7.1)**.[7]

DIAGNOSIS OF INJURY

Cervical esophagus

Suspicion of esophageal injury must be much higher in penetrating than in blunt neck trauma. Clinical examination is quite reliable, as recently shown by large institutional[8] and multicenter studies of 453 asymptomatic patients with no missed injuries.[9,10] In clinical practice, most patients with pharyngoesophageal injuries will have at least some subtle symptoms but can be difficult to assess due to associated injuries and altered sensorium or emotional state, making extensive use of investigations prudent. Indeed, a study by Weigelt showed that clinical examination alone would miss 3 out of 10 cases of esophageal injuries.[11] Signs and symptoms to look out for are neck pain, dysphagia, and sometimes hematemesis and hemoptysis.[12,13] Subcutaneous emphysema can be associated with laryngeal, pharyngeal, tracheobronchial as well as esophageal injuries, but also merely with air entering the tissues from the wound or a pneumothorax. Therefore, it needs to be investigated further with either plain or contrast films, or a CT scan.

Thoracic esophagus

Radiological and endoscopic investigations play a greater role than physical examination in excluding thoracic esophageal injuries. These injuries are more likely to be caused by gunshot or shotgun wounds than by stab wounds, and therefore are mostly associated with injuries to surrounding structures, such as the spine and aorta.[14]

Physical examination is of very little value, other than in the uncommon scenarios of obvious saliva or food draining into a chest tube. There may be abdominal tenderness or rigidity, cervical subcutaneous emphysema on palpation and auscultation (Hamman sign), or nothing specific at all.[14]

Abdominal esophagus, stomach and duodenum

Patients with penetrating injuries to the intra-abdominal esophagus and stomach will usually have signs of peritonism or peritonitis, mainly due to the low pH of gastric juices, and therefore may demonstrate earlier symptoms than those with penetrating injuries of the small or large bowel.[15] Blood from the nasogastric tube is highly suggestive of injury but may be either coming from traumatic insertion or be completely absent, due to food in the stomach, which frequently blocks gastric tubes. Duodenal injuries can be initially asymptomatic, especially if affecting the retroperitoneal portion of the duodenum.[16,17]

INVESTIGATIONS

Failure to repair esophageal injuries within a few hours results in mediastinitis, multiple relooks, and possible death.[18] Mortality rates are calculated at approximately 20–30%, particularly in the thoracic esophagus. For this reason, a high index of suspicion must be entertained when interpreting contrast studies and endoscopy findings. Areas of bruising and localized edema at endoscopy often hide a perforation, and surgery is indicated even for unconvincing signs, in view of what is at stake. Investigations include multiple detector computed tomography (MDCT), contrast swallow studies, and flexible endoscopy with the proviso that injuries may be missed even with a combination of these.[3,19]

Multiple detector computed tomography

This is likely to be the initial investigation in a stable patient, since it can delineate missile tracts, gives a good idea about proximity to vascular and aerodigestive structures and makes further studies and surgery unnecessary by excluding injuries or conclusively proving perforations based on trajectory and abnormalities. It can exclude obvious extravasation and pooling of contrast, if combined with a swallow study, as recently demonstrated by Inaba and colleagues.

Contrast studies

Contrast esophagography is particularly helpful in excluding leaks from the thoracic and abdominal esophagus in alert patients who can swallow. It is less accurate in the cervical esophagus, and in intubated and immobilized patients. Care must be taken to exclude posterior perforations from gunshot wounds close to fractured vertebrae.[20]

Hyperosmolar water-soluble contrast such as gastrografin should be avoided because of the risks of aspiration into the bronchial tree, especially if a concomitant tracheobronchial injury is suspected. A dilute solution of a water-soluble contrast agent such as Omnipaque is preferable, although in resource-poor countries dilute barium solution may still be used. If any doubt persists, a flexible endoscopy should be performed. The negative predictive value of the two modalities combined approaches 100% even with a reported positive predictive value of only approximately 33%.

Endoscopy

Flexible endoscopy is indicated in all suspected injuries of the cervical esophagus, and most suspected injuries in other segments. It may be performed even once the patient is on the operating table for exploratory surgery, in order to avoid missing other injuries and to guide the exposure. It is often difficult to identify an esophageal injury during exploration due to hematomas, bubbling from tracheal injuries and extensive blood staining of the tissues.[14] The advantage of intraoperative esophagoscopy derives from the ability to occlude the distal esophagus and distend the area of suspected injury with air. Care must be taken to avoid missing perforations causing an acute tracheoesophageal fistula, affecting the adjacent walls of esophagus and trachea, which prevent distension of the esophagus. The use of methylene blue has been advocated, but the staining it causes makes further tissue identification and surgery more difficult.

Laparoscopic and thoracoscopy

Thoracoscopy is rarely indicated in the evaluation of thoracic esophageal injuries, in view of the extensive dissection needed to identify penetrating injuries among the extensive damage to surrounding structures. Diagnostic laparoscopy is useful as a screening investigation to look for penetration into the peritoneal cavity, and can identify distal esophageal,ced gastric, and duodenal injuries.[21,22]

INCISIONS AND PROCEDURES

Trauma to the esophagus still results in significant mortality of approximately 20–30%. Morbidity is also extremely high, up to 66%, and independently associated with delay in operative treatment, higher-grade esophageal injury, and the need for resection and the creation of diversion.[23] Important principles of operative surgery are noted below.

Neck

Positioning of the neck in opposite rotation and hyperextension is facilitated by using an air-filled empty intravenous bag, which can then be emptied rapidly at the end of the procedure to facilitate tissue closure.

In suspected penetrating injuries of the cervical esophagus, the initial incision is left anterolateral, over the belly of the sternomastoid muscle, which is then retracted posteriorly, but both sides may need to be explored particularly for transverse trajectories. After cutting through platysma, division of the superior belly of the omohyoid muscle will allow exposure of the proximal carotid sheath, which is then retracted laterally. The common carotid artery and internal jugular vein should be identified and looped, particularly in cases where preoperative radiological investigations were not done, since unsuspected vascular injuries may present, and uncontrolled bleeding or air embolism can be prevented.

A large-bore (32–40 Fr) orogastric tube is inserted by the anesthetist, while the surgeon guides it through the esophagus into the stomach, which is likely to be full. This large tube is kept in during subsequent esophageal repair, and is only replaced by a standard size naso- or orogastric tube for drainage and feeding toward the end of the procedure. After carefully separating the trachea away from the esophagus, avoiding injury to the recurrent laryngeal nerves, the esophagus is encircled by a soft wide drain for traction to facilitate gentle dissection into the posterior mediastinum.[20]

Chest

The incision of choice for a suspected injury of the thoracic esophagus is a right posterolateral thoracotomy, through the fourth, fifth, or sixth intercostal spaces; division of the azygos vein will reveal the esophagus and the carina at that level. Once the esophagus is freed from the densely adherent parietal pleura, its lack of serosal cover and natural flimsiness becomes apparent. For these reasons, buttressing the repair, wide drainage, antibiotics, well-secured gastric tube, and enteral feeding access are crucial.

The most import technique to address the lack of serosal covering is buttressing of the esophageal repair. This can be done with healthy muscle flaps using a two intercostal-wide strip of intercostal tissue, or sternomastoid muscle in the most proximal part of the esophagus. The use of a rhomboid muscle passed into the chest through a separate incision after separation from the nonfeeding-vessel surface of the scapula has also been described. Buttressing is probably not necessary in all cases, but is mainly used in combined tracheal and esophageal injuries or extensive esophageal injuries.[23]

Intra-abdominal esophagus

The identification of injuries of the intra-abdominal esophagus may be very difficult, in view of its intercrural position, which makes for a narrow window, and the presence of possible coexisting bleeding injuries. Extra exposure can, however, be obtained by the widening of the hiatus; and if necessary, radial division of the diaphragm, entering the left pleural cavity, and separating the lower thoracic esophagus away from the descending aorta. Afterwards, any repair should be reinforced with a gastric wrap or a posteriorly based diaphragmatic pedicle.[23] As in other segments, the presence of a large (36–40 Fr) gastric tube, or the use of a Maloney boogie will allow for easier identification and repair.[24]

REPAIR TECHNIQUES

There are several important factors that impact on the outcome of esophageal repairs:
- The esophagus lacks a serosal covering.
- There are sphincters at its proximal and distal ends with subsequent increases in intraluminal pressure.
- There is no redundant length to make up for tissue loss.
- Postrepair gastric tubes may lead to gastroesophageal reflux.
- Dislodgement or early removal a nasogastric tube may prevent adequate feeding.

For the above reasons, early repairs must be meticulous in all cases with careful surgical precision. Interrupted sutures should be used, but individual surgeons may prefer a single- or double-layer technique. Suturing of esophageal injuries must be transverse in the case of small injuries and longitudinal, if longer than 2–3 cm, since the esophagus is difficult to mobilize.

In damage control situations, both external drainage (using a penrose or silastic tube drain) and endoluminal drainage (using a T-tube) may be life-saving.[25]

One must consider a feeding jejunostomy in high-risk repairs, leaving the stomach untouched in case it needs to be used as a conduit or a patch in case of esophageal break down. Surgeons should have a low threshold for postoperative imaging and/or re-exploration in view of the high-risk of leaks. In the longer term, complications such as esophageal stenosis, tracheoesophageal fistula, and chronic infection are relatively common.

Delayed and destructive injuries

Even a delay of 24–48 hours is enough to reduce the success of esophageal repair significantly. In the neck, breakdown may be associated with both attempts at primary suture and the use of a T-tube to obtain a controlled fistula. Loop esophagectomies are very difficult to create, tend to retract, and are more difficulty to control that cervical esophageal fistulas.[26] The consequences of complications in the neck include localized sepsis, a prolonged period of salivary drainage, healing with strictures, but ultimately overall survival is good.

Delays in the thoracic esophagus have far more serious consequences with a high-death rate due to sepsis.[18] Leakage within the thoracic cavity is more difficult to control since mediastinitis may result. Technically, the esophagus itself is very difficult to dissect off the thickened parietal pleura, which may need to be excised in order to access the esophagus. Extensive drainage is necessary, but even then, a difficult thoracic esophagectomy may become necessary, if the mediastinal sepsis does not settle.

Use of esophageal stents

While esophageal stenting for iatrogenic perforation and strictures is widespread, there are very few reports of the use of a stent in penetrating injuries of the esophagus. In the acute setting, early repair is preferred, while in delayed interventions, the whole of the esophagus can be friable and more prone to rupture.

Stenting has been used in occasional cases of traumatic tracheoesophageal fistulas with good results, but only in the thoracic esophagus. The risk of migration distally is also a lot greater because the body of the esophagus is of normal diameter and can expand and lead to dislodgement.[24,27]

Gastric injuries

Investigations

Gastric injuries may be suspected with penetrating thoracic and abdominal injuries. Gastric perforations are almost exclusively due to penetrating trauma,[28] since blunt trauma is more likely to cause a perforation of the small bowel than of the thick-walled stomach.[15]

Pain from gastric perforations is likely to be immediate and more intense than pain from small or large-bowel injuries, due to leakage of acidic gastric contents.

Radiological investigations

Free intraperitoneal air may be seen on plain X-rays, while free intraperitoneal fluid on ultrasound scan is nonspecific.[29] Subtle perforations, especially near the gastroesophageal junction, along the lesser curvature and in the lesser sac may be missed even on double-contrast CT scan[30,31] in view of the frequent plugging of gastric holes by solid food, and variable distension of the stomach by gastrografin. A high index of suspicion is therefore always indicated, based on trajectory and systemic symptoms.[32-35]

The AAST Organ Injury Scale in penetrating trauma related to lacerations can be adapted for the stomach as follows, with one extra grade for multiple injuries up to Grade 3[6] **(Table 7.2)**.

Surgical treatment

A three-dimensional view of the upper abdomen should be obtained by dividing the falciform ligament and ligamentum teres all the way to the diaphragm. Good retraction is essential for adequate exposure and a variety of self-retaining retractors are commercially available.

Table 7.2: American Association for the Surgery of Trauma (AAST) Organ Injury Scale–Lacerations–Stomach.

Grade 1	Partial thickness, not into lumen, serosal tear
Grade 2	*Laceration*: • <2 cm at the gastroesophageal junction or pylorus Or • <5 cm in proximal one-third stomach Or • <10 cm in distal two-thirds stomach
Grade 3	*Laceration*: • >2 cm at the gastroesophageal junction or pylorus Or • 5 cm in the proximal one-third stomach Or • >10 cm in the distal two-thirds stomach
Grade 4	Tissue loss or devascularization <two-thirds stomach
Grade 5	Tissue loss or devascularization >two-thirds stomach

Full decompression of the stomach should be carried out in order to facilitate mobilization and allow inspection of the posterior wall, and allow access to the left upper quadrant. Unfortunately, even large-bore nasogastric tubes are often too small to remove bulky stomach contents, and therefore 36–40 Fr stomach washout tubes or chest drains placed through the mouth by the anesthetist may be needed. Once the stomach is empty, a standard naso- or orogastric tube is placed far into the stomach, so that the greater curvature can be used as a retractor. Injuries close to the gastroesophageal junction are easy to miss, with catastrophic consequences.[36,24] The use of curved soft bowel clamps is very useful in order to allow in insufflation of one segment at a time as may be done in other segments of the GIT. This technique is particularly useful in injuries from sharpened screw drivers, but most importantly for shotgun pellets[32] and shrapnel from explosions,[33,35] since a lot of air may need to be insufflated to identify multiple pinhole perforations throughout the bowel.

Gastric wounds often cause a lot of bleeding, due to the stomach's prolific blood supply, and it is mandatory to incorporate at least a thin edge of mucosa in the suture line. This can be single layer, double layer, or stapled with a GIA™ stapler and thick staples. A combination of Gambee and a few Connell sutures will have the effect of being hemostatic, picking up all the layers and invaginating the mucosa.

If simple repair is not adequate, for example due to severe trauma from explosions and high-energy gunshot wounds, it may be necessary to perform some form of partial or even total gastrectomy. Similar attention to surgical hemostatic technique should be employed.

Most penetrating gastric injuries from grade 1–3 can be sutured in layers, grade 4 may need a partial gastrectomy with or without a Roux-en-Y, and grade 5 may need a total gastrectomy.[37] Areas requiring particular attention are the prepyloric area, the lesser curvature and the vagus nerve, and the short-gastric vessels and the spleen. Care must also be taken while dividing the attachments of the greater curvature to address a very high injury at the posterior gastroesophageal junction.

Damage control surgery requires control of bleeding and contamination. Stapling off blind ends and leaving them inside is not usually appropriate for the stomach and therefore prompt full thickness suturing or GIA stapling is preferable. The restoration of continuity in the setting of damage control is generally reserved for the relook procedure at 24–48 hours.

Duodenum

Injuries of the duodenum can be difficult to manage because of its intimate relation with the pancreas, with frequently combined injuries and management guidelines.[38] This chapter will deal only with isolated duodenal injuries, as it is a very demanding portion of the upper GIT. There are a number of anatomical features, which make the duodenum difficult to assess clinically and to treat:

- It is mainly retroperitoneal, except for the anterior wall of the first part and a very small fourth part, just before the ligament of Treitz, so peritoneal signs may be lacking.
- The posteromedial wall of the first and second part is intimately related to the common bile duct and the main and accessory pancreatic ducts, and cannot be mobilized and sutured with impunity.
- It shares most of its blood supply with the pancreas, originating mainly from the gastroduodenal, superior mesenteric and splenic arteries, which leads to a profuse blood supply and extensive bleeding when injured.
- The second portion is at high-risk of ischemia from arterial injuries to the head of the pancreas, from which its end arteries originate.

In view of its fixed retroperitoneal position, the presence of air, ill-defined masses, and localized retroperitoneal fluid in the right upper posterior abdomen after penetrating trauma are highly suggestive of duodenal injuries, and surgery can be planned accordingly.

The AAST Organ Injury Scale in penetrating trauma for lacerations related to the duodenum is as follows[39] **(Table 7.3)**.

Approach to the duodenum

Duodenal injuries are frequently identified at laparotomy by biliary discoloration in the right upper quadrant, and can be normally packed and ignored initially while bleeding and contamination from other organs are dealt with. In damage control situations, when planning to staple off the small or large bowel and leave the ends inside, or when temporary shunting of vessels is performed, it is better to just leave a drain to the duodenopancreatic injured area rather than trying to repair a badly lacerated duodenum in a hurry. Babcock forceps, clips, and staplers should not be applied to duodenal perforations as a temporary measure, as they will cause damage which may compromise a subsequent primary repair.[40]

Table 7.3: American Association for the Surgery of Trauma (AAST) Organ Injury Scale–Lacerations–Duodenum.	
Grade 1	Partial thickness, not into lumen, serosal tear
Grade 2	Into lumen, <50% of diameter
Grade 3	*Disruption of*: • 50–75% of D2 Or • 50–100% of D1, D3, and D4
Grade 4	*Disruption of*: • >75% of diameter of D2 • Ampulla and distal common bile duct involved
Grade 5	Massive disruption of pancreaticoduodenal structures

Exposure starts with the right colon, avoiding injury to the right ureter, continues with an extended Kocher maneuver, until the inferior vena cava (IVC) and the anterior aspect of Gerota's fascia are well exposed. The duodenum should be inspected for any lacerations on the exposed areas, and then dissection should continue along the inferior aspect of the duodenum proceeding toward the ligament of Treitz. The grade of the injuries identified will then guide toward the various treatment options.[40,41] The method of choice for any individual case should allow for tension and stricture free repair.

Grade 1 laceration—serosal tear

There is no strong evidence for suturing serosal tears, but the fact that the duodenum may become distended and in close proximity to drains makes it prudent to suture the seromuscular layer.

Grade 2 laceration—intraluminal penetration

After debridement to healthy bowel wall, primary repair should be attempted, if a transverse or possibly an oblique suture line is possible. Longitudinal suture lines should be avoided as they are more likely to cause a stricture, which should be avoided in most cases with adequate mobilization.[16,17] The area must be drained with soft non- or low-suction drains, away from the suture line.

Grade 3 and 4 major lacerations

High grades of duodenal injuries are generally, but not always, associated with other serious injuries in the region, and pancreatic, ductal or portal injuries are likely to have a major influence on outcome. These are the injuries for which procedures such as pyloric exclusion and diverticulization were first described.[42,43]

There are a number of useful procedures with which trauma surgeons should be familiar. Those at the more complex end of the scale are rarely performed procedures but can be invaluable in the more challenging cases.[44,45]

- *Graham omental patch*: Simple but hazardous, since it can cause even more duodenal stenosis in the duodenum than in a prepyloric position (15%).
- *Thal patch*: Jejunal loop serosa sutured accurately over the duodenal suture line, with a second layer added to ensure it does not get torn away by weight and gravity.
- *Gallbladder patch*: If an intact and healthy gallbladder is present, it can be mobilized, the tip opened, and sutured around the duodenal defect, at least as a temporizing measure.
- *Pyloric exclusion*: It is the mainstay of treatment for difficult but not devastating duodenal injuries. It consists of the following steps:[46]
  - Repair of the duodenal injury as best as possible.
  - Draining gastrostomy close to the pylorus.
  - Placement of a purse string of absorbable or nonabsorbable suture around the mucosa of the pylorus, taking good bites.
  - Performance of a gastrojejunostomy, preferably retrocolic since the abdomen is likely to be left open, relooks may need to be done, and all suture lines should be as deep as possible within the open abdomen.
  - Drainage of the closed loop of duodenum, either through an intraluminal T-tube, which creates a small controlled fistula; or through a second nasoduodenal tube, down the gastrojejunostomy and passed close to the duodenal repair during surgery. There is debate, as to whether the gastroenterostomy should be closed in due course, lest

it predisposes to junctional peptic ulceration. The consensus is that this is probably not necessary since the gastroenterostomy will become almost nonfunctional, once the duodenal injury has healed and the pylorus is reopened. This may happen either spontaneously or if the suture is cut endoscopically.
- *Roux-en-Y duodenojejunostomy*: This entails the division of the duodenum below the common bile duct and the pancreatic ducts, and an anastomosis of the proximal limb of the duodenum to a jejunal Roux-en-Y.
- Controlled fistulas, acceptable for the first 24–48 hours in damage control, are a last resort for devastating injuries, which do not affect the pancreatic head and therefore do not require a pancreaticoduodenectomy.

Grade 4 and 5 destructive injuries

In many cases of destructive penetrating duodenal injuries, the pancreaticoduodenectomy has already been done by the bullet, and there is little no duodenum left, along with a free hanging common bile duct and badly damaged head of pancreas. In the acute setting, the antrum or the proximal duodenum should be stapled off along with the remaining part of the distal duodenum. Similarly, the common bile duct should be tied off, and a drain inserted adjacent to the pancreas as part of damage control management. Within 24–48 hours, after intensive care unit (ICU) resuscitation, the patient should be taken back to the operating theater for formalization of the Whipple pancreaticoduodenectomy in keeping with institutional protocols and together with hepato-pancreato-biliary (HPB) surgeons.[44]

In all these complex injuries, a feeding jejunostomy should be inserted downstream to allow for enteral feeding for what may prove to be a considerable period of time, particularly in the event of leaks or other significant complications.

CONCLUSION

In summary, penetrating injuries to the duodenum range from a small hole in a portion of the small bowel to destructive retroperitoneal injuries requiring major surgery with input from HPB surgeons. Whatever the case, common sense, sound general surgical skills, generous use of drains, and avoidance of heroic surgery is likely to get the best results.

> **Key points for clinical practice**
> - Penetrating injuries to the upper GIT are likely to present challenges for general surgeons.
> - The esophagus and the duodenum are unforgiving structures with poor tissue qualities and laxity.
> - Anatomy might be distorted by hematomas, presence of a surgical airway, and possibly the need to operate without turning the head because of spinal injuries.
> - The incisions require good planning, are large, and often entail a bilateral neck exploration for cervical esophageal injuries, a right posterolateral thoracotomy with a double lumen tube for the thoracic esophagus, and sometimes the addition of a T extension to a midline laparotomy for complex duodenal injuries.
> - Nonoperative management of minor lower pharyngeal and esophageal injuries has been advocated[47] but has not transferred into practice in the majority of hospitals not exposed to large numbers of penetrating esophageal trauma.[48] Endoscopic interventions may help in selected cases.[49]

- Decisions must be taken early since mortality increases markedly after 24 hours, particularly for thoracic esophageal injuries.[50]
- Buttressing esophageal perforations in the chest can be difficult because of flimsy and traumatized tissues, hence the suggestion to use a wide intercostal pedicle.
- Most duodenal injuries respond well to simple suturing, but the suture line should be protected with a pyloric exclusion, if concerned.
- Good drainage can be life-saving in severe pancreaticoduodenal injuries, and definitive surgery can be planned and performed later.

REFERENCES

1. Vassiliu P, Baker J, Henderson S, et al. Aerodigestive injuries of the neck. Am Surg. 2001;67(1):75-9.
2. Trauma ACOSCO. ACS Advanced Trauma Life Support, 9th edition. American College of Surgeons: Chicago, IL; 2012.
3. Inaba K, Branco BC, Menaker J, et al. Evaluation of multidetector computed tomography for penetrating neck injury: a prospective multicenter study. J Trauma. 2012;72(3):576-83.
4. Shiroff AM, Gale SC, Martin ND, et al. Penetrating neck trauma: a review of management strategies and discussion of the 'no zone' approach. Am Surg. 2013;79(1):23-9.
5. Richardson JD. Management of oesophageal perforations: the value of aggressive surgical treatment. Am J Surg. 2005;190(2):161-5.
6. Tisherman SA, Bokhari F, Collier B, et al. Clinical practice guideline: penetrating zone II neck trauma. J Trauma. 2008;64:1392-405.
7. Moore EE, Jurkovich GJ, Knudson MM, et al. Organ injury scaling. VI: extrahepatic biliary, oesophagus, stomach, vulva, vagina, uterus (nonpregnant), uterus (pregnant), fallopian tube, and ovary. J Trauma. 1995;39(6):1069-70.
8. Demetriades D, Theodorou D, Cornwell E, et al. Evaluation of penetrating injuries of the neck: prospective study of 223 patients. World J Surg. 1997;21(1):41-7.
9. Asensio JA, Chawan S, Forno W, et al. Penetrating oesophageal injuries: Multicenter study of the American Association for the Surgery of Trauma. J Trauma. 2001;50(2):289-96.
10. Neville A. Penetrating injuries to the pharynx and cervical oesophagus. In: Velmahos GC, Degiannis E, Doll D (Eds). Penetrating Trauma, 2nd edition. Springer: Verlag, Berlin Heidelberg, DE; 2017.
11. Weigelt JA, Thal ER, Snyder WH, et al. Diagnosis of penetrating cervical oesophageal injuries. Am J Surg. 1987;154(6):619-22.
12. Teixeira F, Menegozzo CA, Netto SE, et al. Safety in selective surgical exploration in penetrating neck trauma. World J Emerg Surg. 2016;11:32.
13. Biffle W, Moore EE, Feliciano DV, et al. Western Trauma Association Critical Decisions in Trauma: diagnosis and management of oesophageal injuries. J Trauma Acute Care Surg. 2015;79(6):1089-95.
14. Ivatury RR, Leppaniemi A, Biffle W, et al. Oesophageal injuries: position paper, WSES, 2013. World J Emerg Surg. 2014;9(1):9.
15. Rodrigues-Hermosa JI, Roig J, Sirvent JM, et al. Gastric perforations from abdominal trauma. Dig Surg. 2008;25(2):109-16.
16. Snyder WH 3rd, Weigelt JA, Watkins WL, et al. The surgical management of duodenal trauma. Precepts based on a review of 247 cases. Arch Surg. 1980;115(4):422-9.
17. Timaran CH, Martinez O, Ospina JA. Prognostic factors and management of civilian penetrating duodenal trauma. J Trauma. 1999;47(2):330-5.
18. Asensio JA, Berne J, Demetriades D, et al. Penetrating oesophageal injuries: time interval of safety for preoperative evaluation—how long is safe? J Trauma 1997;43(2):319-24.
19. Mirvis SE. Imaging of acute thoracic injury: the advent of MDCT screening. Semin Ultrasound CT MR. 2005;26(5):305-31.
20. Sperry JL, Moore EE, Coimbra R, et al. Western Trauma Association critical decisions in trauma: penetrating neck trauma. J Trauma Acute Care Surg. 2013;75(6):936-40.
21. Carrillo EH, Heniford BT, Etoch SW, et al. Video-assisted thoracic surgery in trauma patients. J Am Coll Surg. 1997;184(3):316-24.

22. Shan CX. Is laparoscopy equal to laparotomy in detecting and treating small bowel injuries in a porcine model? World J Gastroenterol. 2012;18(46):6850-5.
23. Richardson JD, Tobin GR. Closure of oesophageal defects with muscle flaps. Arch Surg. 1994;129(5):541-8.
24. Schellenberg M, Inaba K, Bardes JM, et al. Defining the gastroesophageal junction in trauma: Epidemiology and management of a challenging injury. J Trauma Acute Care Surg. 2017;83(5):798-802.
25. O'Connor JV, DuBose JJ, Scalea TM. Damage-control thoracic surgery: management and outcomes. J Trauma Acute Care Surg. 2014;77(5):660-5.
26. Dasari B, Neely D, Kennedy A, et al. The role of oesophageal stents in the management of oesophageal anastomotic leaks and benign oesophageal perforations. Ann Surg. 2014;259(5):852-60.
27. Blackmon, Shanda H, Schwarz P, et al. Utility of removable oesophageal covered self-expanding metal stents for leak and fistula management. Ann Thorac Surg. 2010;89(3):931-7.
28. Velmahos GC, Demetriades D, Toutouzas KG, et al. Selective nonoperative management in 1,856 patients with abdominal gunshot wounds: should routine laparotomy still be the standard of care? Ann Surg. 2001;234(3):395-403.
29. Rozycki GS, Ballard RB, Feliciano DV, et al. Surgeon-performed ultrasound for the assessment of truncal injuries: lessons learned from 1540 patients. Ann Surg. 1998;228(4):557-67.
30. Phillips T. Use of the contrast-enhanced CT enema in the management of penetrating trauma to the flank and back. J Trauma. 1986;26(7):593-601.
31. Goodman CS, Hur JY, Adajar MA, et al. How well does CT predict the need for laparotomy in hemodynamically stable patients with penetrating abdominal injury? A review and meta-analysis. Am J Roentgenol. 2009;193(2):432-7.
32. Flint LM, Cryer HM, Howard PA, et al. Approaches to the management of shotgun injuries. J Trauma. 1984;24(5):415-9.
33. Almogy G, Mintz Y, Zamir G, et al. Suicide bombing attacks: can external signs predict internal injuries? Ann Surg. 2006;243(4):541-6.
34. Champion HR. Injuries from explosions: physics, biophysics, pathology, and required research focus. J Trauma. 2009;66(5):1468-77.
35. Bala M, Rivkind AI, Zamir G, et al. Abdominal trauma after terrorist bombing attacks exhibits a unique pattern of injury. Ann Surg. 2008;248(2):303-9.
36. Kawahara N, Alster C, Fujimura I, et al. Standard examination system for laparoscopy in penetrating abdominal trauma. J Trauma. 2009;67(3):589-95.
37. Chavarria-Aguilar M, Cockerham WT, Barker DE, et al. Management of destructive bowel injury in the open abdomen. J Trauma. 2004;56(3):560-4.
38. Lopez PP, Benjamin R, Cockburn M, et al. Recent trends in the management of combined pancreatoduodenal injuries. Am Surg. 2005;71(10):847-52.
39. Moore EE, Cogbill TH, Malangoni MA, et al. Organ injury scaling, II: Pancreas, duodenum, small bowel, colon, and rectum. J Trauma. 1990;30(11):1427-9.
40. Mayberry J, Fabricant L, Anton A, et al. Management of full-thickness duodenal laceration in the damage control era: evolution to primary repair without diversion or decompression. Am Surg. 2011;77(6):681-5.
41. Jansen M, Du Toit DF, Warren BL. Duodenal injuries: surgical management adapted to circumstances. Injury. 2002;33(2):611-5.
42. Seamon MJ, Pieri PG, Fisher CA, et al. A ten-year retrospective review: does pyloric exclusion improve clinical outcome after penetrating duodenal and combined pancreaticoduodenal injuries? J Trauma. 2007;62(4):829-33.
43. Talving P, Nicol AJ, Navsaria PH. Civilian duodenal gunshot wounds: surgical management made simpler. World J Surg. 2006;30(4):488-94.
44. Delcore R, Stauffer JS, Thomas JH, et al. The role of pancreatogastrostomy following pancreatoduodenectomy for trauma. J Trauma. 1994;37(3):395-400.
45. Velmahos GC, Kamel E, Chan LS, et al. Complex repair for the management of duodenal injuries. Am Surg. 1999;65(10):972-5.
46. Degiannis E, Krawczykowski D, Velmahos GC, et al. Pyloric exclusion in severe penetrating injuries of the duodenum. World J Surg. 1993;17(6):751-4.
47. Madiba TE, Muckart DJ. Penetrating injury to the Cervical Oesophagus: is routine exploration mandatory? Ann R Coll Surg Eng. 2003;85(3):162-6.

48. Petrone P, Kassimi K, Jimenez-Gomez M, et al. Review: management of esophageal injuries secondary to trauma. Injury. 2017;48(8):1735-42.
49. Sudarshan M, Elharram M, Spicer J, et al. Management of esophageal perforation in the endoscopic era: is operative repair still relevant? Surgery. 2016;160(4):1104-10.
50. Aiolfi A, Inaba K, Demetriades D, et al. Non-iatrogenic esophageal injury: a retrospective analysis from the National Trauma Data Bank. World J Emerg Surg. 2017;12:19.

Section 6

Lower Gastrointestinal Surgery

CHAPTERS

8. Novel Radiotherapy Techniques for the Treatment of Anal Cancer
9. Anorectal and Perineal Manifestations of Tuberculosis
10. Surgical Considerations during Pregnancy and Delivery in Women with Crohn's Disease

Chapter 8

Novel radiotherapy techniques for the treatment of anal cancer

Paul Shaw, Rhydian Maggs

INTRODUCTION

There are approximately 1,300 new cases of anal cancer (**Figure 8.1**) in the United Kingdom annually, representing less than 1% of all new cancer cases (2014). More than half (52%) of anal cancer cases in the United Kingdom are diagnosed in people aged over 65 but the incidence rates are highest in people aged 85–89 (2012–2014). The incidence rate of anal cancer has risen by 56% since the early 1990s, with the largest increase being in females (almost 90% increase), compared to an increase of 17% for males. It is projected that the incidence of anal cancer is set to rise by 43% between 2015 and 2035 to 4 cases per 100,000 people by 2035. It is estimated that 1 in 795 men and 1 in 470 women will be diagnosed with anal cancer during their lifetime. Anal cancer is more common in deprived regions. Over the last decade anal cancer mortality rates have remained stable for both sexes. Current UK statistics for 2014 reveal 140 male and 220 female anal cancer deaths with 48% occurring in people aged 75+ (2012–2014). The 1-, 5- and 10-year survival rates for anal cancer in England are 86%, 64% and 57% respectively, being similar for men and women (http://www.cancerresearchuk.org/health-professional/cancer-statistics/statistics-by-cancertype/anal-cancer#heading-Three).

Many factors determine the risk of developing cancer including age, genetics, environmental and lifestyle factors. It is estimated that 90% of anal cancers are linked to lifestyle and other risk factors. The most significant potentially avoidable risk factor is human papillomavirus (HPV) infection which is thought to be linked to 90% of cases in the United Kingdom. Human immunodeficiency virus (HIV) infection increases the risk of anal cancer, but evidence is lacking to classify the risk of anal cancer linked to smoking, organ transplantation and vulval or cervical precancerous lesions (http://www.cancerresearchuk.org/health-professional/cancer-statistics/statistics-by-cancer-type/anal-cancer#heading-Three).

ROLE OF SURGERY IN THE TREATMENT OF ANAL CANCER

Although chemoradiotherapy is now standard first line practice, surgery continues to have an important role in the local excision of well-differentiated tumors less than 2 cm in diameter providing that clear surgical margins can be obtained and anal sphincter function preserved. Abdominoperineal resection (APR) is now seldom the primary treatment, but may be indicated in patients where pelvic radiation is contraindicated (e.g. previous radiation or transplanted kidney). It is important to recognize that APR does not treat the

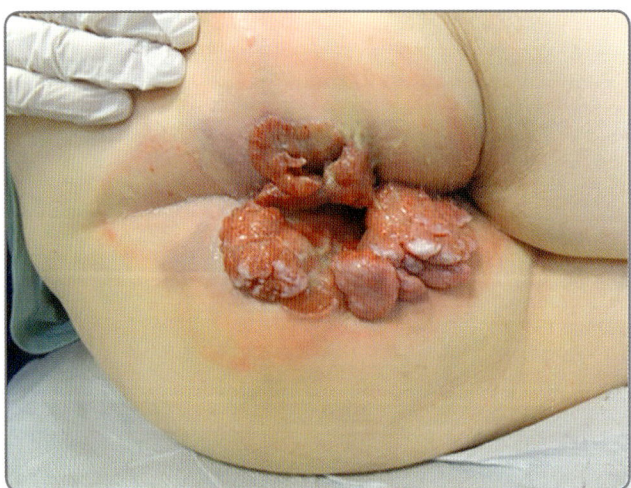

Figure 8.1 T3N3 basaloid squamous anal tumor extending to the perianal tissues.

pelvic lymph nodes which are at risk of micrometastatic spread. Surgical expertise is also required for defunctioning loop colostomy in the presence of bulky symptomatic tumors, fecal incontinence or where there is evidence of fistulization.

ROLE OF CHEMORADIOTHERAPY IN THE TREATMENT OF ANAL CANCER

The role of radiation and chemotherapy was first recognized in the 1970s when Nigro et al. delivered a preoperative chemoradiation schedule. The dose schedule delivered 30 Gy in 15 fractions with two cycles of chemotherapy [5-fluorouracil (5-FU) and mitomycin C] and 7 of 12 patients had no viable tumor evident in the postoperative specimen.[1,2] In the 1990s, the UKCCR published the ACT1 trial including 585 patients, demonstrating improved local failure rates of combined chemotherapy with radiation.[3] However, this was associated with significantly greater toxicity compared with radiation alone due in part to the large nonconformal radiation fields used at this time. Building on this trial ACT2, the largest randomized trial in anal cancer to date, has reaffirmed 5-FU and mitomycin with 50.4 Gy radiation in 28 daily fractions as the standard of practice.[4] With median follow-up of 5.1 years, 90% of patients achieve complete response at 26 weeks and 3-year progression-free survival of 73%. The most common grade 3–4 toxic effects experienced by patients were skin damage (47%), pain (29%), hematological suppression (16%) and gastrointestinal (GI) toxicity (18%)). Radiation continues to be combined with mitomycin and 5-FU or oral capecitabine in line with NCCN and ESMO guidance (http://www.tri-kobe.org/nccn/guideline/colorectal/english/anal.pdf).[5] Neoadjuvant or adjuvant cisplatin/5-FU chemotherapy have not demonstrated improvements in outcome.[6]

RADIATION TOXICITY

Radiation for anal cancer was historically delivered using large orthogonal volumes which did not conform to the internal anatomy of patients and thus delivered excess dose to normal

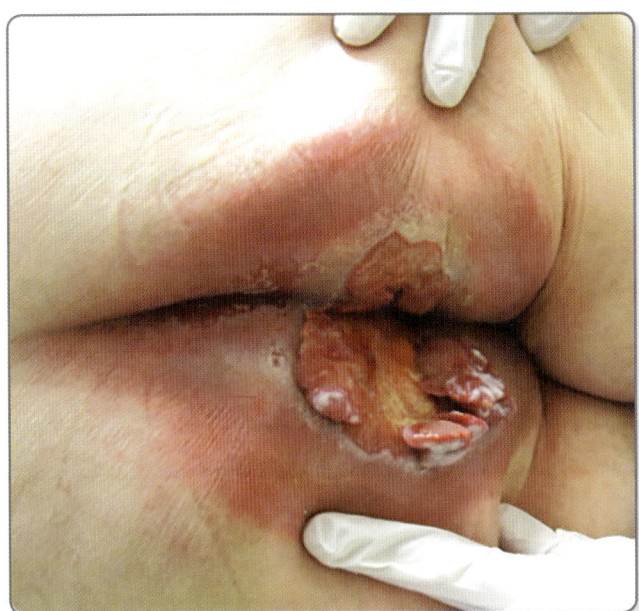

Figure 8.2 Acute radiation toxicity seen after 3 weeks of radiation delivered to patient with T3N3 anal tumor.

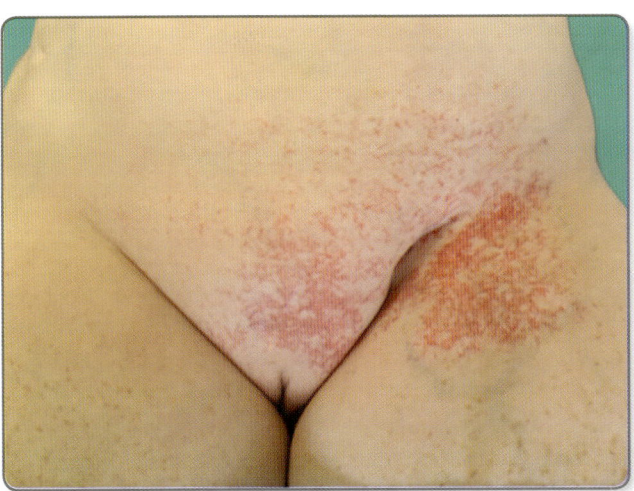

Figure 8.3 Late effects of radiation from conventional three-dimensional (3D) conformal radiation resulting in marked skin telangiectasia.

tissues which contributed to toxicity, tolerance and outcome. This resulted in significant acute and chronic toxicity to the skin of the perineum, perianal areas and upper thighs (**Figures 8.2 and 8.3**).

CONTOURING RADIATION VOLUMES

Computed tomography (CT), magnetic resonance imaging (MRI) and positron emission tomography-CT (PET-CT) are used to identify the target regions to be treated. These, together

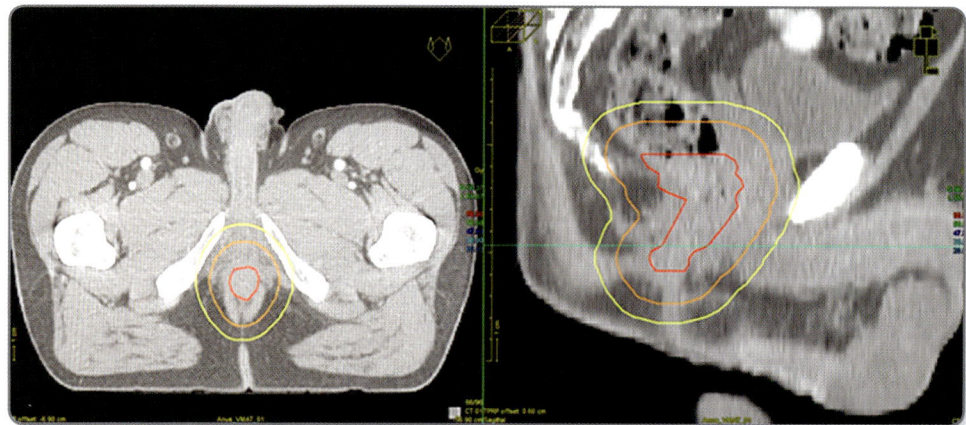

Figure 8.4 Cross-sectional CT imaging to demonstrate creation of treatment volumes in anal cancer. Gross tumor volume (red contour), clinical target volume (orange contour) and planning target volume (yellow contour).

with clinical examination alongside examination under anesthesia, inform delineation of gross tumor volumes (GTVs) on a CT scan performed in the treatment position. Target generation is performed in stages—the GTV is defined as the palpable tumor and to this a margin is added to account for subclinical spread to derive the clinical target volume (CTV). Further geometric margins are added to account for target motion and patient setup uncertainty to yield the planning target volume (PTV) to which it is intended to deliver the prescription dose. Several PTVs may be defined for treatment to different dose levels depending on the nature of the target volume (e.g. macroscopic/microscopic disease) (**Figure 8.4**).

DEVELOPMENTS IN RADIOTHERAPY TECHNIQUES

Technical advances have enabled radiation to be delivered to anal tumors and their draining lymph node regions with greater precision by incorporating advances in diagnostic imaging (CT, MRI, PET-CT imaging) alongside improvements in radiation dose distribution, including dose intensification and accurate delivery. These novel techniques include intensity-modulated radiation therapy (IMRT) and volume-modulated arc therapy (VMAT). IMRT and VMAT are now standard of care approaches for radiation delivery in anal cancers to enhance the dose modeling of radiation toward the tumor target(s) and in favor of protecting normal tissues, with the added potential for dose escalation.

ADVANCED RADIOTHERAPY DELIVERY METHODS

Intensity-modulated radiation therapy and VMAT are advanced radiotherapy delivery techniques which allow precise tailoring of doses to the target volume. IMRT beams are delivered from static positions around the patient but the intensity of radiation across the fields is modulated using multileaf collimators (MLCs) to preferentially shield or expose different portions of the field over the entire field delivery. Similarly, VMAT uses the MLCs to modulate the field intensity but the radiation is delivered continuously as the beam rotates around the patient. Both methods have the advantage of allowing the high doses to be closely conformed to complex target shapes and deliver different dose levels within a single plan. This allows for reduction in doses to healthy tissues and specifically delineated organs at risk (OARs) without compromising target coverage. Further potential benefits may include the opportunity to escalate doses to targets beyond conventional prescriptions. VMAT delivery is generally quicker than both conventional and IMRT. Disadvantages of these methods include an increased volume of healthy tissue receiving a low dose, which has the potential to increase the possibility of inducing secondary malignancies—highlighting the importance of selecting appropriate patients for these techniques. The advent of these advanced techniques has been possible thanks to improvements in processing ability and software to allow for the very complex treatments to be optimized. Typically, the time and resource to produce these plans is much greater than for conventional conformal radiation therapy (RT), but this is improving **(Figure 8.5)**.

With more precise target definition and greater conformality of RT plans, there is a requirement for greater precision of patient setup verification during treatment. The introduction of cone beam CT (CBCT) as an imaging modality to the clinic has allowed for three-dimensional (3D) imaging at the time of treatment, and verification of the position of the delivered doses with respect to the soft tissue targets. A further advantage of this system is that it provides data to allow for adaptive planning to account for patient shape changes compared to the original planning scan, whereby modifications are made to the RT plan to take account for these patient variations. There is however additional RT dose from these interventions, so this must be carefully balanced against the benefits.

Guidance for the implementation of IMRT for anal cancer has been developed.[7] Phase II evaluation of IMRT in combination with 5-FU and mitomycin[8] has demonstrated a

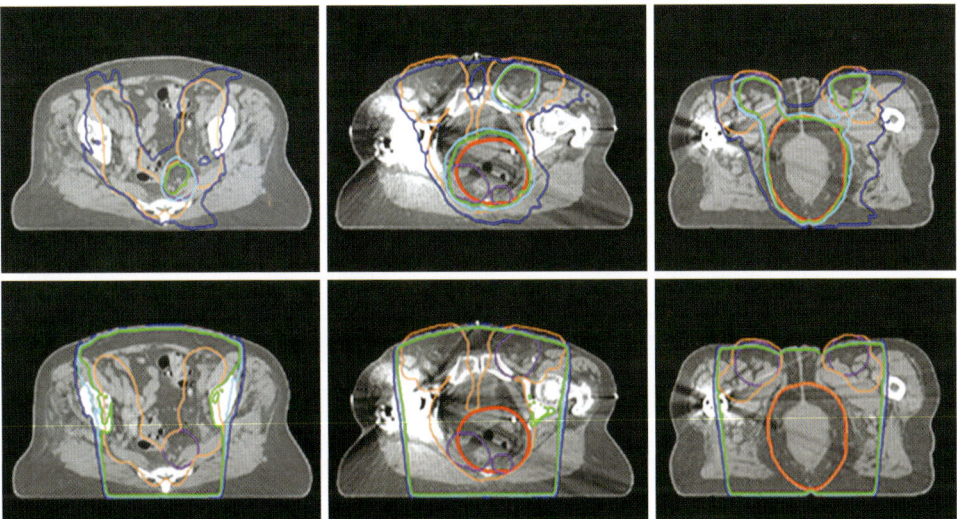

Figure 8.5 Improved radiation dose distribution with volume modulated arc therapy (VMAT). The upper panel demonstrates greater conformality between the target volume (green) and the 95% radiation isodose line (blue) and the ability to deliver differential dose distributions to a complex volume using VMAT. In comparison, the lower panel shows that a less conformal radiation field increases the doses to normal tissues. In this example, the dose to the small bowel has been significantly reduced with conformal VMAT treatment.

significant reduction in grade 3 skin, GI and grade 2 hematological events. Grade 3 GI toxicity was 21% compared with historical rates of 36% reported in Radiation Therapy Oncology Group (RTOG) 9811 with conventional radiation fields; genitalia and inguinal regions were spared significant grade 3 skin toxicity (23% vs 49%). In a retrospective analysis of conformal radiation using 3-5 static fields versus VMAT[9] conventional conformal radiation resulted in a systematic failure to achieve ideal radiotherapy dose volume objectives whereas VMAT reduced the radiation doses to bladder, bowel and genitals. In this study, VMAT reduced the incidence of higher grade toxicity and grade 2-3 toxicity was reduced by 20% (GI); 6% [genitourinary (GU)] and 7% (skin). A National Audit of Anal Cancer Radiotherapy[7] has shown that many patients now receive IMRT or equivalent delivery (78%) and is associated with lowered acute toxicity (ACT2 trial 71% vs IMRT 48%). The main reductions in acute toxicity relate to grade 3 and 4 skin toxicity (40% vs 25%).

There is a lack of published data regarding the late toxic effects of radiation using anal IMRT. A retrospective study of 27 evaluable anal cancer patients receiving IMRT has recently reported baseline profiles of outcomes related to bowel and sexual dysfunction. Over 3 years observation points, questionnaire scores for bowel symptoms [inflammatory bowel disease questionnaire (IBDQ), illness behaviour questionnaire (IBQ-B) and Vaizey incontinence scores] were stable or improving, and showed good bowel continence for most patients. Treatment was reported to affect sexual relationships in 3/6 (50%) males and 2/21 (10%) females.[10] Psychosexual effects of radiation are likely to be a significant cause of morbidity and concern for some patients.

Reported outcome measures differ between different anal cancer trials and such measures may also be weighted differently by both patients and clinicians in terms of their importance. A recent initiative (CORMAC) is inviting patients, clinicians and trialists to define which outcomes should be included in a core outcome set. This will help to reduce the heterogeneity limiting future trial comparisons and endorse the value of variables measured.

BRACHYTHERAPY

Intensity-modulated radiation therapy/VMAT with daily imaging guidance to ensure correct delivery to target is expected to reduce radiation dose to OARs of damage, lead to reductions in acute toxicity and might facilitate radiation dose escalation. An alternative approach to this may be provided by integrating brachytherapy to boost dose to the primary disease in patients with locally advanced disease (e.g. T3/4). Brachytherapy is highly conformal radiation delivery to small volumes and in anal cancer can be used to boost the dose to the primary tumor whilst limiting the dose to surrounding normal structures. Although high-dose rate brachytherapy greater than 12 Gy/hour is the most frequent technique, an alternative approach would be interstitial implantation of radioisotopes. To enable sphincter preservation brachytherapy should be restricted to anal tumors that extend to less than 50% circumference, less than 5–10 mm thickness and less than 5 cm in the craniocaudal plain. In anal cancer, the majority of cases treated with brachytherapy have received this treatment 2–3 weeks after external beam radiotherapy (EBRT), noting that the overall treatment time and interval between EBRT and brachytherapy are prognostic indicators of local control.[11]

PROTON BEAM THERAPY

Proton beam therapy is likely to become a treatment modality in the future for anal cancers, with US centers offering this capability presently. Protons are deposited at a defined depth

(Bragg peak) which is dependent upon beam energy level with the potential advantage of targeting escalated radiation doses more accurately to the tumor with greater avoidance of surrounding normal tissues compared to photons. Proton beam IMRT may produce highly conformal treatments with reduced hematological toxicity associated with prophylactic nodal volumes.[12]

ANAL CANCER TRIALS

Future trials need to be as efficient as possible, especially in the setting of rare diseases where patient numbers are small. To tackle this, an umbrella trial (PLATO) developed in the United Kingdom is recruiting patients with anal cancer to examine several important questions:
- Selective chemoradiation after local excision of anal margin tumors
- Reduced dose chemoradiation to primary anal tumors in order to reduce late effects whilst maintaining prophylactic nodal irradiation in early-stage disease
- Dose-escalated chemoradiation in locally advanced T3/4 N+ stage disease.

The international multicenter PLATO (personalising anal cancer radiotherapy dose) study, umbrella trial will consist of ACT3, ACT4 and ACT5 trials. ACT3 is an nonrandomized phase study (n = 90) which will examine the strategy of local excision for T1N0 anal margin tumors with selective postsurgical chemoradiation for involved fields and concurrent capecitabine for patients with margins less than or equal to 1 mm. ACT4 will randomize (n = 162) patients in a phase II setting to either reduced dose chemoradiation with 41.4 Gy in 23 fractions or 50.4 Gy in 28 fractions to the anal primary tumor using concurrent capecitabine for T1/2 (<4 cm) N0 stage disease. ACT5 will evaluate (n = 677) patients in a seamless pilot (n = 60), phase II (n = 140) and subsequent phase III study to compare dose escalated radiotherapy to the primary cancer with either 5-FU or capecitabine in late stage T3/4 N+ disease. The primary endpoints for each trial will be locoregional failure at 3 years.[13]

OTHER ANAL CANCER TRIALS: TARGETED AGENTS/ IMMUNOTHERAPY IN COMBINATION WITH RADIATION

Strategies to attempt improved treatment outcomes for anal cancer patients have examined enhancing the effects of locally delivered radiation with combined novel anticancer therapeutics. Approaches have, for example, included antagonism of cancer cell survival signals [e.g. epidermal growth factor receptor (EGFR) signaling] with the use of combined anti-EGFR monoclonal antibodies with radiation. More recent developments in the field of immuno-oncology have naturally led to interest extending to combinations with radiation given that radiotherapy may enhance tumor antigen exposure to the immune system.

A phase II study examining the role of cetuximab, a monoclonal antibody targeting EGFR in 62 patients treated with chemoradiation (cisplatin-5-FU) plus 8 weekly cetuximab demonstrated a modest improvement in 3-year locoregional failure (20% compared with historical rates of 35%), but at the expense of significant (32%) grade 4 toxicity including life-threatening events (1 death).[14] Panitumumab has also been combined with mitomycin and 5-FU and radiation in squamous cell anal cancer[15] with results in abstract form suggesting that this regimen may be more tolerable, although outcome data is awaited.

Evidence is accumulating that radiation is an immune stimulus, recruiting immune mediators that enable antitumor responses both within and beyond radiation fields. A body of evidence is developing that supports the combination of immunotherapies with radiation on the basis that irradiated tumor, through induction of immunogenic cell death and damping down of an immunosuppressive tumor microenvironment, is able to act as an in situ vaccine, to enhance both local and systemic anticancer effects.[16] The combination of immunotherapy with radiation is likely to be reflected in future anal cancer trials. Current work in the field of immunology also includes examining the role of ADXS11-001 to stimulate the immune system against HPV-infected anal cancer cells in combination with standard chemoradiation for anal cancer.

METASTATIC ANAL CANCER TRIALS

The InterAACT study aims to provide the first randomized evidence for the treatment of inoperable locally recurrent and metastatic squamous cell carcinoma of the anus to identify the optimal chemotherapy backbone treatment (cisplatin/5-FU vs carboplatin/paclitaxel). This will also guide which standardized chemotherapy should be combined with targeted agents in future studies and to confirm the feasibility of conducting an international multicenter trial for this rare tumor.[17]

The immune check point inhibitor nivolumab, a monoclonal antibody targeting the programmed cell death-1 (PD-1) receptor on T cells (to promote immune cell attack of T cells against HPV-positive cells) has been examined in refractory metastatic squamous cell cancer of the anus in a phase II study. Among 37 patients evaluable, 9 (24%) had responses. There were 2 complete responses and 7 partial responses. Grade 3 adverse events were anemia (n = 2), fatigue (n = 1) and rash (n = 1). No serious adverse events were reported and may represent a future promising treatment.[18] Pembrolizumab is also being examined in this setting.

> **Key points for clinical practice**
>
> - Anal cancer incidence is increasing.
> - Current standard treatment is definitive chemoradiation incorporating concurrent 5-FU/mitomycin chemotherapy.
> - Newer methods of radiotherapy such as IMRT and VMAT can reduce toxicity whilst achieving equivalent clinical benefit.
> - Current anal cancer trials are looking at the role of radiotherapy, including radiation dose enhancement and de-escalation in defined clinical situations.
> - Targeted drug and immunotherapy combinations will likely influence future radiation trials in anal cancer.
> - Survivorship issues relating the anal cancer treatment will to continue to be an ongoing focus of care.

REFERENCES

1. Nigro ND, Vaitkevicius VK, Considine B Jr. Combined therapy for cancer of the anal canal: a preliminary report. Dis Colon Rectum. 1974;17(3):354-6.
2. Nigro ND, Seydel HG, Considine B, et al. Combined preoperative radiation and chemotherapy for squamous cell carcinoma of the anal canal. Cancer. 1983;51(10):1826-9.

References

3. Epidermoid anal cancer: results from the UKCCCR randomised trial of radiotherapy alone versus radiotherapy, 5-fluorouracil, and mitomycin. UKCCCR Anal Cancer Trial Working Party. UK Co-ordinating Committee on Cancer Research. Lancet. 1996;348(9034):1049-54.
4. James RD, Glynne-Jones R, Meadows HM, et al. Mitomycin or cisplatin chemoradiation with or without maintenance chemotherapy for treatment of squamous-cell carcinoma of the anus (ACT II): a randomised, phase 3, open-label, 2 × 2 factorial trial. Lancet Oncol. 2013;14(6):516-24.
5. Glynne-Jones R, Nilsson PJ, Aschele C, et al. Anal cancer: ESMO-ESSO-ESTRO clinical practice guidelines for diagnosis, treatment and follow-up. Radiother Oncol. 2014;111(3):330-9.
6. Ajani JA, Winter KA, Gunderson LL, et al. Fluorouracil, mitomycin, and radiotherapy vs fluorouracil, cisplatin, and radiotherapy for carcinoma of the anal canal: a randomized controlled trial. JAMA. 2008;299(16): 1914-21.
7. Muirhead R, Drinkwater K, O'Cathail SM, et al. Initial results from the Royal College of Radiologists' UK National Audit of Anal Cancer Radiotherapy 2015. Clin Oncol (R Coll Radiol). 2017;29(3):188-97.
8. Kachnic LA, Winter K, Myerson RJ, et al. RTOG 0529: a phase 2 evaluation of dose-painted intensity modulated radiation therapy in combination with 5-fluorouracil and mitomycin-C for the reduction of acute morbidity in carcinoma of the anal canal. Int J Radiat Oncol Biol Phys. 2013;86(1):27-33.
9. Tozzi A, Cozzi L, Iftode C, et al. Radiation therapy of anal canal cancer: from conformal therapy to volumetric modulated arc therapy. BMC Cancer. 2014;14:833.
10. Francesco D, Thomas K, Wedlake L, et al. Intensity-modulated radiotherapy and anal cancer: clinical outcome and late toxicity assessment. Clin Oncol. 2016;28(9):604-10.
11. Glynne-Jones R, Tan D, Hughes R, et al. Squamous-cell carcinoma of the anus: progress in radiotherapy treatment. Nat Rev Clin Oncol. 2016;13(7):447-59.
12. Intensity modulated proton therapy is being investigated in a clinical study determine if the dose of radiation to normal tissues can be reduced (NCT03018418).
13. Sebag-Montefiore D, Adams R, Bell S, et al. The development of an umbrella trial (PLATO) to address radiation therapy dose questions in the locoregional management of squamous cell carcinoma of the anus. Int J Radiat Oncol Biol Phys. 2016;96(2):E164-5.
14. Garg MK, Zhao F, Sparano JA, et al. Cetuximab plus chemoradiotherapy in immunocompetent patients with anal carcinoma: a Phase II Eastern Cooperative Oncology Group-American College of Radiology Imaging Network Cancer Research Group Trial (E3205). J Clin Oncol. 2017;35(7):718-26.
15. Feliu J, Garcia-Carbonero R, Capdevila J, et al. Phase II trial of panitumumab (P) plus mytomicin C (M), 5-fluorouracil (5-FU), and radiation (RT) in patients with squamous cell carcinoma of the anal canal (SCAC): safety and efficacy profile—VITAL study, GEMCAD 09-02 clinical trial. J Clin Oncol. 2014;32:5.
16. Kang J, Demaria S, Formenti S. Current clinical trials testing the combination of immunotherapy with radiotherapy. J Immunother Cancer. 2016;4:51.
17. Sclafani F, Adams RA, Eng C, et al. InterAACT: an international multicenter open label randomized phase II advanced anal cancer trial comparing cisplatin (CDDP) plus 5-fluorouracil (5-FU) versus carboplatin (CBDCA) plus weekly paclitaxel (PTX) in patients with inoperable locally recurrent (ILR) or metastatic disease. J Clin Oncol. 2015:1-24. http://ascopubs.org/doi/abs/10.1200/jco.2015.33.3_suppl.tps792:
18. Morris VK, Salem ME, Nimeiri H, et al. Nivolumab for previously treated unresectable metastatic anal cancer (NCI9673): a multicentre, single-arm, phase 2 study. Lancet Oncol. 2017;18(4):446-53.

Chapter 9

Anorectal and perineal manifestations of tuberculosis

Arunima Verma, Sunil Kumar

INTRODUCTION

Worldwide, tuberculosis (TB) remains a major cause of morbidity and mortality,[1] but the exact incidence of TB is difficult to ascertain due to incomplete reporting and imprecise diagnostic criteria. However, 14% of newly diagnosed reported cases are extrapulmonary TB[2] and it is estimated that miliary TB accounts for 1-2% of TB cases in immunocompetent individuals.[3] The resurgence of TB, with the HIV pandemics, brought a new spectrum of clinical presentations, and increased incidence of extrapulmonary manifestations mainly involving the lymphatics, urinary, digestive, and central nervous systems.[4-8] Extrapulmonary spread often comprises of involvement of pleura (26%), lymph nodes (17%), genitourinary tract (15%), bones and joints (14%), meninges (6%), peritoneum (4%), and miliary TB (8%).[9,10]

Gastrointestinal (GI) TB is responsible for only 1% of all cases of TB and is the sixth most frequent site of extrapulmonary involvement.[11] Any part of the GI system may be affected. The most common GI manifestation is tuberculous peritonitis and the most frequently affected part is the ileocecal region.[9] In decreasing order, GI localizations include the ileocecal region, the ascending colon, the jejunum, the appendix, the duodenum, the stomach, the esophagus, the sigmoid colon, and the rectum.[12] Spread to the anus is rare and occurs in approximately 0.7% of cases.[13]

Anoperineal TB is more commonly seen in men (4:1 ratio) and in those that practice receptive anal intercourse.[14] It usually starts from the 4th decade.[15] The pediatric population has a greater incidence of anal TB compared to adults.[16] Although extrapulmonary TB is common among HIV-positive patients,[17] it seems that the incidence of perianal involvement is not increased by HIV infection.[18]

PATHOGENESIS

Perianal TB usually coexists with a pulmonary lesion or may develop by reactivation of the latent focus.[18,19] Approximately, 20-25% of GI TB cases present with concomitant pulmonary TB.[20] There are various pathogenetic mechanisms described for the development of perianal TB. Ingestion of airway secretions containing high amounts of *Mycobacterium tuberculosis* bacilli and, sometimes, inoculation or ingestion of contaminated milk or food may lead to anal contamination. The incidence of contaminated milk is rare nowadays due to pasteurization of milk. Tubercle bacilli can also reach the perianal region by hematogenous spread from the primary lung focus in childhood where it may be reactivated to cause anal

Box 9.1: Pathogenesis of perianal tuberculosis.

- Ingestion of *Mycobacterium tuberculosis* bacilli
- Hematogenous spread
- Direct spread from contiguous organs
- Via lymphatic channels from infected nodes

Box 9.2: Clinical features of perianal tuberculosis.

- Anorectal sepsis
- Anal ulceration with inguinal lymphadenopathy
- Fistula-in-ano
- Anal fissure
- Hemorrhoidal nodules
- Perianal cutaneous tubercular lesions (e.g. lupus vulgaris, tuberculosis verrucosa cutis)
- Rectal stricture (short, annular, and firm with nodular surface)
- *Others*—pilonidal sinus, rectal submucosal tumor, recurrent perianal lesions, and other atypical presentations

TB (**Box 9.1**). Direct spread from adjacent organs and spread through lymph channels from infected nodes have also been postulated.[6,7,21-23]

CLINICAL PRESENTATION AND MANIFESTATIONS (BOX 9.2)

Clinical signs and symptoms may mimic malignancy or Crohn's and it is only after biopsy that diagnosis is confirmed. Rectal TB is a rare presentation of abdominal TB with presenting features being hematochezia (88%), constitutional symptoms (75%), constipation (37%), and rarely fistula.[24] The most common anal manifestation of TB is usually multiple fistulae and 14% of fistula-in-ano are tubercular in some geographical areas.[25] Most cases present with anal discharge and perianal swelling is found only in one-third. Since TB causes obliterative endarteritis, obliterative endarteritis, massive bleeding is not a feature of colonic TB, but massive hematochezia in rectal TB does occur due to mucosal trauma caused by the scybalous stool traversing the stricturous segment. Tuberculous skin lesions of the perianal and anorectal regions may present as part of GI or genitourinary TB. Bacon et al. classified perianal TB into four types[26] as shown in **Table 9.1**.

DIAGNOSIS

Despite the availability of multiple tests, early diagnosis of anal/perianal TB remains a challenge.[27,28] Both Crohn's and TB have overlapping clinical, radiological, endoscopic, and histologic characteristics.

Demonstration of acid-fast bacilli (AFB) in biopsy specimens or mycobacterial culture is the most specific investigation, but diagnostic yield for these procedures is low especially in cases of extrapulmonary TB.[29-31]

Table 9.1: Classification of perianal tuberculosis.

	Type of lesion	TB type	Manifestation
1	Ulcerative	Pulmonary/GI TB	Superficial ulcerations with hemorrhagic necrotic base and well-defined boundaries
2	Verrucous	*Mycobacterium bovis*	Wart, hemorrhoidal nodules, perianal abscess or fistula
3	Lupoid TB	TB anywhere in body	Nodule, which turns into clean cut ulcer with indurated base and mucopurulent discharge
4	Miliary	Disseminated TB	Involves many organs besides perianal TB

(TB: Tuberculosis; GI: Gastrointestinal).

If there is a clinical suspicion of TB, clinical evaluation with history and physical examination should be done followed by routine tests such as total leukocyte count, erythrocyte sedimentation rate, Mantoux test, microscopy, and culture for AFB in the discharge from the lesion or tissue section from the lesion. Radiological imaging and molecular tests may also be useful.

Pulmonary TB should be sought in all cases, as it is present concomitantly in most patients with GI TB. Chest radiography, followed by CT chest if needed, should be done along with a tuberculin skin test and sputum sent for acid-fast smear and culture.

Mantoux test

The tuberculin skin test can be a supportive diagnostic tool, if positive, but a negative skin test does not exclude the diagnosis. In endemic areas, the result of tuberculin skin test alone is not sufficient evidence to diagnose extrapulmonary TB in adult patients.[32] Tuberculin positivity in abdominal TB is 58–100%,[33-37] and in cutaneous TB is 67%,[38] both of which are associated with perianal TB.

Acid-fast smear

Acid-fast bacilli smear microscopy using the conventional light microscope is still the mainstay of diagnosis and monitoring treatment of TB in endemic countries, as it is simple, inexpensive, widely applicable, and highly specific. The sensitivity of direct AFB smear is low and detects AFB only when 10^5 bacilli per mL are present.[39] The efficacy of smear microscopy can be increased by concentration techniques such as Petroff's method and staining by Auramine O (AO) fluorescent dye using light emitting diode (LED) based fluorescent microscopes as against Ziehl–Neelsen (ZN) with conventional or bright field (BF) microscope.[39-41]

Culture for *mycobacterium tuberculosis*

Specimens should be inoculated into culture medium. The standard technique of using solid medium Lowenstein–Jensen (LJ) culture method is time consuming and use of the radiometric BACTEC 460 TB system is faster and more sensitive. Other systems available are MB/BacT, which has lower sensitivity compared to BACTEC 460 TB, especially with smear-negative specimens. The average number of days required for detection of *M. tuberculosis* complex is 15.4 for BACTEC 460 TB, 17.2 for MB/BacT, and 29.8 for LJ medium.[42]

Histopathology

Histopathology of a tissue biopsy specimen in the presence of TB may show TB granulomas, which typically contain epithelioid macrophages, Langhans giant cells, and lymphocytes. Characteristic caseating necrosis seen in the centers of tuberculous granulomas often supports a diagnosis of TB.[25,43]

Radiology

Ultrasonography of abdomen and pelvis, computed tomography (CT) scan of abdomen and pelvis, and magnetic resonance imaging (MRI) of perineum may be used depending upon the presenting symptoms. Ultrasound may reveal multiple echogenic lesions with surrounding hypoechoic halos and CT may demonstrate multiple foci of low attenuation, typically without enhancement after intravenous contrast administration. Thickening of the wall of the colon and terminal ileum is seen along with rectal stricturing. Lymph nodes may be markedly enlarged and are often of low attenuation with necrotic centers and a thick enhancing inflammatory rim. Calcification, fistulae, and sinus tracts may also be seen.[44] In addition, other features of abdominal TB such as ascites, mesenteric infiltration, omental mass, peritoneal enhancement/thickening, and disorganized masses of soft tissue density may also be seen along with granulomas or abscesses in the liver, pancreas, and spleen.[24] CT for anal lesions should probably be limited to the diagnosis of fistula-associated pelvic abscesses where other imaging is unavailable or cannot be tolerated.[45] Transperineal sonography is an inexpensive and easily available diagnostic tool, which may help in detecting a variety of pathological conditions of the lower rectum, the anus, and the perianal region.[46] Anal endosonography has no specific role in the diagnosis of perianal TB, but may be useful in assessing fistula anatomy and sphincter integrity.[45] The possibility of anorectal TB should be considered when MRI pelvis shows extra-sphincteric sinus tracts, multiple external openings, lymphadenopathy, altered marrow, and osteomyelitis of pelvic bones in a patient having recurrent fistula/sinus tracts.[47] Among other imaging, Gallium scan has been found to be a convenient and useful method for evaluating extrapulmonary TB lesions other than TB meningitis and may be used after CT and MRI in selected cases.[48,49]

Endoscopy

Endoscopic differential diagnosis of anorectal TB includes Crohn's disease, herpes simplex lesions, cytomegalovirus, sarcoidosis, amoebiasis, deep mycosis, syphilis, actinomycosis, lymphogranuloma venereum, and ulcerative neoplasms. Many of these conditions have similar features including mucosal ulceration, nodularity, aphthous ulcers, edematous mucosal folds, strictures, pseudopolyps, colonic skip lesions, ileocecal spread, and granulomas on histological examination.[50] Rectal TB can present with annular stricture or with ulceration of mucosa with fibrosis. Its radiological and endoscopic appearances may be extremely similar to malignant rectal lesions and only biopsy can confirm the diagnosis.[51]

Molecular tests

Polymerase chain reaction (PCR) has been used to confirm the diagnosis of cutaneous TB,[52,53] as it is positive in 50–60% of cases as compared to very low positivity by culture. PCR is also useful in cases of lymphadenopathy, which have positivity rates varying from 40 to 90.[54-57]

Rapid immunochromatographic assay (RIA) for the diagnosis of TB may be a valuable adjunct to standard techniques of TB diagnosis. It has a high specificity, even in extrapulmonary TB, and might prove to be a suitable instrument for first-line testing of suspected cases in resource-poor countries where access to diagnostic tools is limited and cost efficiency has a high priority.[58]

When perianal TB is a part of miliary TB, other molecular tests available are nucleic acid amplification assays (NAA) such as amplified *Mycobacterium tuberculosis* direct (MTD) test (Gen-Probe) and Amplicor (Roche) to test sputum or respiratory secretions in pulmonary TB, and Xpert MTB/RIF assay, which is also useful for detection of extrapulmonary TB in lymph nodes and CSF.[59-63]

Flowchart 9.1 shows an algorithm for the diagnosis of suspected anal/perianal TB.

TREATMENT

Once the diagnosis is established, specific medical antitubercular therapy (ATT) is commenced along with surgical treatment of anal manifestations. **Box 9.2** shows clinical manifestations of anal/perianal TB and each would need to be addressed accordingly, e.g. surgical treatment of anal sepsis and surgical removal of fistula and sinuses. Tuberculous fistula or sinuses may heal after ATT, but it is recommended that they should be excised completely, though the tracts are complex, as failure of definitive surgical excision may lead to recurrances.[64] The recommended surgical procedures are usually conservative and are required in the presence of clinical complications such as intestinal obstruction due to anal stenosis or rectal stricture. Anal stenosis may initially be managed conservatively by dilatation but those persisting beyond 6 months of ATT may need surgical treatment in the form of anoplasty. Rectal stricture leading to obstruction would need excision of the strictured segment via anterior resection or abdominoperineal resection (APR). Lesions with coexisting malignancy or mimicking malignancy need surgical excision.[65]

The standard 6-month regimen of ATT consists of an intensive phase of 2 months of isoniazid (INH), rifampin (RIF), pyrazinamide (PZA), and ethambutol (EMB) followed by a continuation phase of 4 months of INH and RIF. In special situations such as HIV-infected patients, those receiving antiretroviral therapy (ART) should be given the standard 6-month regimen and those not receiving ART should have an extended continuation phase with INH and RIF for an additional 3 months.[66]

Key points for clinical practice

- Tuberculosis is a major infectious disease worldwide but anoperineal TB is still an uncommon manifestation of this disease.
- Perianal TB may result from hematogenous, lymphatic, or direct spread from other TB sites.
- Clinical manifestation varies according to the lesion and may mimic other conditions, e.g. malignancy and Crohn's disease.
- Perianal TB is usually four types: (1) ulcerative, (2) verrucous, (3) lupoid, and (4) miliary.
- Culture of *Mycobacterium tuberculosis* from infected tissue or discharge material is the gold standard for diagnosis.
- Radiology, endoscopy, and molecular tests may be used to aid diagnosis in culture-negative cases where index of suspicion is high.
- Once diagnosed, medical treatment with ATT is started and surgical treatment, which is usually conservative, is done according to the clinical manifestation.

Treatment

Flowchart 9.1 Algorithm for diagnosis of anal or perianal lesions suspicious of tuberculosis.

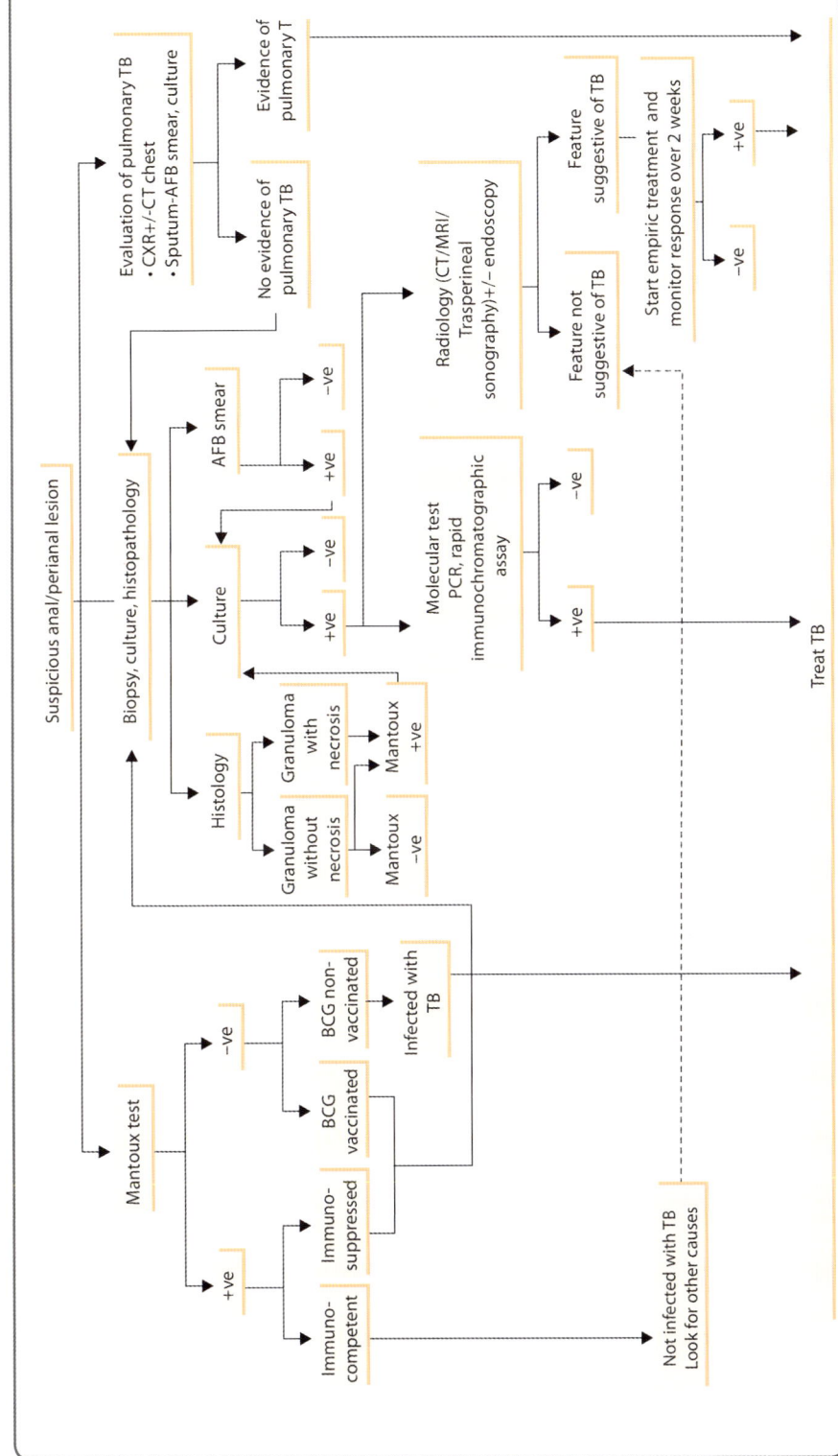

(AFB: Acid-fast bacilli; CT: Computed tomography; MRI: Magnetic resonance imaging; TB: Tuberculosis; PCE: Polymerase chain reaction; BCG: Bacillus Calmette–Guérin).

REFERENCES

1. Baylon SC, Barros MSV, Christiano CG, et al. Rectal tuberculosis in an HIV-infected patient: case report. Autopsy Case Rep. 2014;4(3):65-9.
2. World Health Organization. (2015). Global tuberculosis report 2015. [online] Available from http://www.who.int/tb/publications/global_report/en/. [Accessed September, 2017].
3. Sharma SK, Mohan A, Sharma A, et al. Miliary tuberculosis: new insights into an old disease. Lancet Infect Dis. 2005;5(7):415.
4. Lopes L, Certo M, Ramada J, et al. Tuberculosis intestinal. J Port Gastrenterol #(Portuguese). 2004;11:25-9.
5. Loureiro MP, Cruz P, Fontana A, et al. Tuberculose intestinal- diagnostic e ressecçâo minimamente invasivos. Rev Bras Vídeocir #(Portuguese). 2006;4:13-6.
6. Sá Ribeiro FA, Alves ALF. Doenças inflamatórias e infecciosas. In: Vieira OM, Chaves CP, Manso JEF, Eulálio JMR (Eds). Clinica cirúrgica: fundamentos teóricos e práticos. São Paulo: Atheneu; 2000. pp. 253-8.
7. Grisi SJFE, Cardoso AC, Bellizia L, et al. Tuberculose peritoneal: relato de caso e comparação de métodos diagnósticos. Pediatria (Portuguese). 2001;23:100-5.
8. Chuttani HK, Sarin SK. Intestinal tuberculosis. Ind J Tub. 1985;32:117-25.
9. Mehta JB, Dutt A, Harvil L, et al. Epidemiology of extrapulmonary tuberculosis. A comparative analysis with pre-AIDS era. Chest. 1991;99(5):1134-8.
10. Sbarbaro JA. Tuberculosis in the 1990s. Epidemiology and therapeutic challenge. Chest. 1995;108(2):58-62.
11. Sharma MP, Bhatia V. Abdominal tuberculosis. Indian J Med Res. 2004;120(4):305-15.
12. Marshall JB. Tuberculosis of the gastrointestinal tract and peritoneum. Am J Gastroenterol. 1993;88:989-99.
13. Alvarez Conde JL, Gutierrez Alonso VM, Del Riejo Tomas J, et al. Perianal ulcers of tubercular origin. A report of 3 new cases. Rev Esp Enferm Dig. 1992;81(1):46-8.
14. Ghosh SK, Bandyopadhyay D, Ghosh A, et al. Perianal dermatosis among men who have sex with men: a clinical profile of 32 Indian patients. Dermatol Online J. 2011;17(1):9-11.
15. Ibn Majdoub Hassani K, Ait Laalim S, Toughrai I, et al. Perianal Tuberculosis: A case report and a Review of the Literature. Case Rep Infect Dis. 2012;2012:852763.
16. Bandyopadhyay S. Tuberculosis in Gastroenterology Practice: clinical challenges. Medicine Update. 2011;321-31.
17. Harries AD, Maher D. TB/HIV A Clinical Manual. Geneva: World Health Organization; 1996. pp. 46-60.
18. Sultan S, Azria F, Bauer P, et al. Anoperineal tuberculosis: diagnostic and management considerations in seven cases. Dis Colon Rectum. 2002;45(3):407-10.
19. Akgun E, Tekin F, Ersin S, et al. Isolated perianal tuberculosis. Neth J Med. 2005;63(3):115-7.
20. Pujari BD. Experience with tuberculosis of the large bowel. Indian J Surg. 1989;51:57-64.
21. Horland RW, Varkey B. Anal tuberculosis: report of two cases and literature review. Am J Gastroenterol. 1992;87(10):1488-91.
22. Addison NV. Abdominal tuberculosis—a disease reviewed. Ann Royal Coll Surg Engl. 1983;65(2):105-11.
23. Gupta J. Anoperineal tuberculosis—solving a clinical dilemma. Af Health Sci, 2005;5(4):345-7.
24. Bandyopadhyay S, Das C, Maity PK, et al. Isolated colonic tuberculosis with colovesical fistula. J Assoc Physicians India. 2010;58:396.
25. Shukla HS, Gupta SC, Singh C, et al. Tubercular fistula-in-ano. Br J Surg. 1988;75:38-9.
26. Nepomuceno OR, Grady JFO, Eisenberg SW, et al. Tuberculosis of the anal canal: report of a case. Dis Colon Rectum. 1971;14(4):313-6.
27. Le Bourgeois PC, Poynard T, Modai J, et al. Peri-anal ulceration. Tuberculosis should not be overlooked. Presse Medicale. 1984;13(41):2507-9.
28. Chung CC, Choi CL, Kwok SPY, et al. Anal and Perianal tuberculosis: a report of three cases in 10 years. J Royal Coll Surg Edinb. 1997;42(3):189-90.
29. Samarasekera DN, Nanayakkara PR. Rectal tuberculosis: A rare cause of recurrent rectal suppuration. Colorectal Dis. 2008;10(8):846-7.
30. Haldar S, Chakarvorty S, Bhalla M, et al. Simplified detection of Mycobacterium tuberculosis in sputum using smear microscopy and PCR with molecular beacons. J Med Microbiol. 2007;56(Pt 10):1356-62.
31. Kiraz N, Akgun LEY, Kasifoglu N, et al. Rapid detection of Mycobacterium tuberculosis from sputum specimens using the FAST Plaque TB test. Int J Tuberc Lung Dis. 2007;11(8):904-8.
32. Sharma SK, Mohan A. Extrapulmonary tuberculosis. Indian J Med Res. 2004;120:316-53.
33. Singh MM, Bhargava AN, Jain KP. Tuberculosis peritonitis: an evaluation of pathogenic mechanisms, diagnostic procedures and therapeutic measures. N Engl J Med. 1969;281(20):1091-4.
34. Singh V, Jain AK, Agrawal AK, et al. Clinicopathological profile of abdominal tuberculosis. Br J Clin Pract. 1995;49(1):22-4.

35. Manohar A, Simjee AE, Haffejee AA, et al. Symptoms and investigative findings in 145 patients with tuberculous peritonitis diagnosed by peritoneoscopy and biopsy over a five-year period. Gut. 1990;31(10): 1130-2.
36. Szmigielski W, Venkatraman B, Ejeckam GC, et al. Abdominal tuberculosis in Qatar: a clinico-radiological study. Int J Tuberc Lung Dis. 1998;2(7):563-8.
37. Balasubramanian R, Nagarajan M, Balambal R, et al. Randomised controlled clinical trial of short course chemotherapy in abdominal tuberculosis: a five-year report. Int J Tuberc Lung Dis. 1997;1(1):44-51.
38. Kumar B, Muralidhar S. Cutaneous tuberculosis: a twenty-year prospective study. Int J Tuberc Lung Dis. 1999;3(6):494-500.
39. Hooja S, Pal N, Malhotra B, et al. Comparison of Ziehl Neelsen and Auramine O staining methods on direct and concentrated smears in clinical specimens. Indian J Tuberc. 2011;58(2):72-6.
40. Munshi SK, Rahman F, Mostofa Kamal SM, et al. Comparisons among the diagnostic methods used for the detection of extra-pulmonary tuberculosis in Bangladesh. Int J Mycobacteriol. 2012;1:190-5.
41. Zaib-un-Nisa, Javed H, Zafar A, et al. Comparison of fluorescence microscopy and Ziehl-Neelsen technique in diagnosis of tuberculosis in paediatric patients. J Pak Med Assoc. 2015;65(8):879-81.
42. Roggenkamp A, Hornef MW, Masch A, et al. Comparison of MB/BacT and BACTEC 460 TB systems for recovery of mycobacteria in a routine diagnostic laboratory. J Clin Microbiol. 1999;37(11):3711-2.
43. Candela F, Serrano P, Arriero JM, et al. Perianal disease of tuberculous origin: report of a case and review of the literature. Dis Colon Rectum. 1999;42:110-2.
44. Thoeni RF, Cello JP. CT Imaging of Colitis. Radiology. 2006;240(3):623-38.
45. Halligan S, Stoker J. Imaging in Fistula-in-ano. Radiology. 2006;239:18-33.
46. Bonatti H, Lugger P, Hechenleitner P, et al. Transperineal sonography in anorectal disorders. Ultraschall Med. 2004;25(2):111-5.
47. Naphade PS, Raut AA, Kulkarni VM, et al. (2010). Anorectal tuberculosis: MR imaging spectrum. ECR 2010. [online] Available from www.myesr.org. [Accessed September, 2017].
48. Lin WY, Hsieh JF. Gallium-67 citrate scan in extrapulmonary tuberculosis. Nuklearmedizin. 1999;38(6):199-202.
49. Yang SO, Lee YI, Chung DH, et al. Detection of extrapulmonary tuberculosis with gallium-67 scan and computed tomography. J Nucl Med. 1992;33(12):2118-23.
50. Santra G, Pani A, Biswas K. Isolated rectal tuberculosis with multiple ulcers. J Assoc Phys India. 2013;61(12): 934-6.
51. Puri AS, Vij JC, Kumar N, et al. Diagnosis and outcome of isolated rectal tuberculosis. Dis colon Rectum. 1996;39(10):1126-9.
52. Arora SK, Kumar B, Sehgal S. Development of a polymerase chain reaction dot blotting system for detecting cutaneous tuberculosis. Brit J Dermatol. 1999;142(1):1-6.
53. Margall N, Baselga E, Coll P, et al. Detection of Mycobacterium tuberculosis DNA by the polymerase chain reaction for rapid diagnosis of cutaneous tuberculosis. Br J Dermatol. 1996;135:231-6.
54. Narayanan S, Parandaman V, Rehman F, et al. Comparative evaluation of PCR using IS 6110 and a new target in the detection of tuberculous lymphadenitis. Curr Sci. 2000;78:1367-70.
55. Kwon KS, Dh CK, Jang HS, et al. Detection of mycobacterial DNA in cervical granulomatous lymphadenopathy from formalin fixed paraffin embedded tissue by PCR. J Dermatol. 2000;27(6):355-60.
56. Singh KK, Muralidhar M, Kumar A, et al. Comparison of in house polymerase chain reaction with conventional techniques for the detection of Mycobacterial tuberculosis DNA in granulomatous lymphadenopathy. J Clin Pathol. 2000;53(5):355-61.
57. Rimek D, Tyagi S, Kappe R. Performance of an IS 6110-based assay and the COBAS AMPLICOR MTB PCR system for the detection of Mycobacterium tuberculosis complex DNA in human lymph node samples. J Clin Microbiol. 2002;40(8):3089-92.
58. Grobusch MP, Schürmann D, Schwenke S, et al. Rapid immunochromatographic assay for diagnosis of tuberculosis. J Clin Microbiol. 1998;36(11):3443.
59. Panel on Opportunistic Infections in HIV-Infected Adults and Adolescents. (2017). Guidelines for the prevention and treatment of opportunistic infections in HIV-infected adults and adolescents: recommendations from the Centers for Disease Control and Prevention, the National Institutes of Health, and the HIV Medicine Association of the Infectious Diseases Society of America. [online] Available from http://aidsinfo.nih.gov/contentfiles/lvguidelines/adult_oi.pdf. [Accessed September, 2017].
60. Havlir DV, Barnes PF. Tuberculosis in patients with human immunodeficiency virus infection. N Engl J Med. 1999;340(5):367.

61. Vadwai V, Boehme C, Nabeta P, et al. Xpert MTB/RIF: a new pillar in diagnosis of extrapulmonary tuberculosis? J Clin Microbiol. 2011;49(7):2540.
62. Tortoli E, Russo C, Piersimoni C, et al. Clinical validation of Xpert MTB/RIF for the diagnosis of extrapulmonary tuberculosis. Eur Respir J. 2012;40(2):442.
63. Denkinger CM, Schumacher SG, Boehme CC, et al. Xpert MTB/RIF assay for the diagnosis of extrapulmonary tuberculosis: a systematic review and meta-analysis. Eur Respir J. 2014;44(2):435.
64. Gupta PJ. Ano-perianal tuberculosis—solving a clinical dilemma. Afr Health Sci. 2005;5(4):345-7.
65. Patil S, Shah AG, Bhatt H, et al. Tuberculosis of rectum simulating malignancy and presenting as rectal prolapse—a case report and review. Indian J Tuberc. 2013;60(3):184-5.
66. Nahid P, Dorman SE, Alipanah N, et al. Official American Thoracic Society/Centers for Disease Control and Prevention/Infectious Diseases Society of America Clinical Practice Guidelines: treatment of drug-susceptible tuberculosis. Clin Infect Dis. 2016;63(7):e147-95.

Chapter 10

Surgical considerations during pregnancy and delivery in women with Crohn's disease

Faris Soliman, Rachel Hargest

INTRODUCTION

Crohn's disease (CD) is one of the two most common forms of inflammatory bowel disease (IBD), named after Dr Burrill B Crohn who was part of the team to first describe the condition.[1-3] Adverse outcomes in pregnancy have been shown to be higher in patients with IBD.[4] Therefore, the challenges facing women with CD during their reproductive years may require specialist expertise and input, in order to allow conception and maintain pregnancy through to delivery while ensuring safety and minimizing potential complications to the mother and baby. There are several misconceptions surrounding pregnancy in potential mothers with CD, both within the population and amongst medical staff, which can affect and influence choices for patients with CD, particularly given that limited evidence is currently available.

FECUNDITY AND FERTILITY

It has been shown that between 50% and 70% of patients with CD will require surgery within 5 years of diagnosis.[5] Patients with IBD have fewer children than the general population, both reflecting voluntary childlessness by women, as well as women suffering with active disease.

While women with quiescent CD have fertility equal to the general population, active CD reduces fertility. The reduction in fertility in active CD can occur for a variety of reasons including:
- Pelvic inflammation affecting uterus, fallopian tubes, and ovaries
- Previous surgical intervention
- Active perianal disease causing dyspareunia
- Chronic active disease causing menstrual and hormonal abnormalities
- Voluntary childlessness or reduction in family size.

MULTIDISCIPLINARY STRUCTURE

Two multidisciplinary teams (MDT) overlap in the care of pregnant patients with CD. Both the obstetric MDT and IBD MDT have involvement in management decisions together with the patient.

The obstetric team is made up of obstetricians, midwives, dedicated anesthetists, pediatricians, and labor ward support personnel. The Royal College of Obstetrics and Gynaecology have recommended minimum safe staffing levels at for each of these. It has also been advocated to move to more consultant-led service provision, particularly in busy obstetric centers.

The IBD team structure in the UK has set standards regarding the minimum number of specialists within the multidisciplinary team based on a defined population of 250,000.[3] The team is made up of and includes consultant gastroenterologists and colorectal surgeons, clinical nurse specialists specific to IBD, clinical nurse specialists specific to stoma therapy and ileoanal pouch surgery, gastroenterology-specific dieticians and pharmacists, a nutrition support team, histopathologists, and radiologists. Finally, completing the team structure, administrative support is essential to running an effective MDT.

The IBD MDT should also have access to the wider medical support team for the extraintestinal manifestations of IBD, who have a specific interest in IBD patients. This again includes psychologists/counselors, rheumatologists, ophthalmologists, dermatologists, and consultant pediatricians. Finally, an established link to local community practice is necessary, often through a designated general practitioner (family practitioner), to ensure liaison and education within the community medical practices.

MEDICAL MANAGEMENT PRECONCEPTION

It has been shown that lack of knowledge regarding aspects of pregnancy in patients with CD is associated with negative views around the entire process. A large proportion of patients think that medication is harmful to the fetus and that all medication should be stopped prior to conception and put up with symptoms.[6] Many patients have also been shown to be worried about passing on IBD to offspring, as well the effects of pregnancy on IBD, and vice-versa. A small proportion of patients consider choosing not to conceive due to their worries and lack of information.

It is, therefore, important to tackle these misconceptions early on, even prior to patients considering reproduction, so that when they do attempt to conceive, they seek the correct medical support and guidance in order to maintain disease control and reduce complications during pregnancy.

Aims of preconception management include gaining control of active disease, patient education and adjusting patient medication to reduce the risk of fetal malformation and complication rates.

MEDICAL MANAGEMENT DURING PREGNANCY

If a patient conceives at a time where there is controlled or nonactive disease, the risk of relapse is approximately equal to the risk of relapse in nonpregnant women with CD.[7] However, if conception is at a time of active disease, relapse rates are found to be significantly higher during pregnancy. Pregnancy itself is thought to improve the outcomes of CD with the need for surgery reducing as the pregnancy progresses. It has been observed that mothers who have had a previous pregnancy require fewer surgical interventions during pregnancy than women in their first pregnancy.[8] It is considered that active disease poses the greatest risk to mother and fetus during pregnancy. Nutritional supplementation is an important component, particularly in the first trimester, as the need is increased early in pregnancy.

MEDICATION DURING PREGNANCY

There are misconceptions regarding which medication is safe to use and which medications need to be avoided in patients with CD who are trying to conceive or are pregnant. **Table 10.1** includes a list of key medications used in CD for disease control, together with their safety profile and complications reported in pregnancy. Limited research and data are available and as result options available to the clinician are reduced. **Table 10.2** includes medication used for the symptom management of patients with Crohn's.

Table 10.1: Key medication in Crohn's disease (CD) for disease control.

Drug	
Corticosteroids	• Cross the placental barrier • Considered safe due to the rapid conversion to less active metabolites leading to low fetal blood concentrations • Possible induction of preterm birth[9] • Possible slight increase in risk of cleft palate[10] • Can be used to treat acute flares of disease
Budesonide	• Limited data on the safety of budesonide in pregnancy • Small study looking at its use during pregnancy showed no untoward effect[11]
Aminosalicylates	• Mesalazine thought to be safe • Particularly at doses of <3 g/day[12]
Thiopurines	• Generally considered safe • No significant reports of adverse effects on pregnancy in humans • Extreme doses in animals have caused congenital defects
Cyclosporin	• Most data comes from transplant patients on immunosuppression • Small studies show low-complication rates, with no reported birth malformations • Prematurity, low-birth weight, and spontaneous abortion have been reported
Tacrolimus	• Thought to be safe without causing excess congenital malformation • Associated with premature births
Methotrexate	• Methotrexate should be avoided in pregnancy • Teratogenic and embryotoxic effects • Long half-life • Takes approximately 6 weeks to clear completely
Anti-TNF drugs	• Long-term implications of anti-TNF therapy not known • Use should be considered with caution • Anti-TNF antibodies able to cross the placental barrier in the third trimester • Infliximab and adalimumab have shown no significant increase in the rates of congenital malformation, abortion, or still birth compared to those in the disease control population or the general population[13,14]
Thalidomide	• Absolutely contraindicated in pregnancy • Associated with major fetal abnormalities involving limbs, eyes and ears, neural tube defects, hemangioma, and duodenal fistulae • Neonatal mortality significantly increased

(TNF: Tumor necrosis factor).

Table 10.2: Medication used for symptom control in Crohn's disease (CD).

Drug	
Analgesia	• Paracetamol and codeine are considered safe • Nonsteroidal anti-inflammatory drugs (NSAIDs) not recommended due to limited research
Antidiarrheal	• Loperamide and cholestyramine are considered generally safe
Antiemetics	• Ondansetron and metoclopramide are considered safe
Antacids/H_2 receptor antagonists/proton-pump inhibitors	• Antacids and H_2 receptor antagonists are considered safe • Proton-pump inhibitors used with caution, with a low-teratogenic risk[15,16]
Antibiotics	• Use the shortest possible course • Avoid tetracyclines—skeletal retardation and teeth discoloration • Avoid Sulfonamides—teratogenic due to interference with folic acid metabolism • Avoid metronidazole especially high doses • Most other antibiotics considered safe

SURGERY FOR CROHN'S DISEASE DURING PREGNANCY

Surgery for abdominal Crohn's disease

The indications for surgery in pregnant women with CD are the same as those in nonpregnant women with CD. These include perforation, obstruction, hemorrhage, acutely ischemic bowel, and drainage of unresolved intra-abdominal sepsis, which cannot be drained radiologically. Patients presenting with gastrointestinal fistulae should again be managed in the same way as in nonpregnant patients[17] with the aim of getting mother and baby safely to term. The argument for this approach is that ongoing illness is felt to be a greater risk to the fetus than operative management. The type of surgery required to get the mother and baby out of trouble is dependent on the presenting pathology. Patients should make decisions on management taken in consultation with a gastroenterologist, a colorectal surgeon and an obstetrician.

Non-Crohn's abdominal emergencies, such as incarcerated hernia, perforated peptic ulcer or abdominal trauma should be managed as for any other patient according to basic surgical principles. The best outcome for the baby is likely to occur, if the management of the mother is optimized. Early delivery should be considered, if a surgical emergency or cancer presents at 36+ weeks of pregnancy.

Surgery for perianal Crohn's disease

When considering perianal CD, management of perianal sepsis is important to protect the sphincter complex with regard to continence. Surgery is sometimes needed for uncomplicated perianal fistulae but nearly always needed for complex disease. The simplest form of management is usually abscess drainage with seton placement in the presence of a fistula-in-ano. Sometimes, a defunctioning stoma and rarely a proctectomy are required for patients failing medical therapy. Small studies have shown that combined medical and surgical therapy is superior to either medical or surgical therapy alone.[18-20] Advancement flaps have also been used in the treatment of Crohn's fistulae, but rarely during pregnancy. Newer modalities, such as fistula plugs, glue, and stem cells, have still to be evaluated in the long-term but are rarely licensed for use in pregnancy. Moreover, recurrence rates have been reported to be high.

There is a potential danger that the rarity of acute surgical problems during pregnancy may cause both a delay in referral and in decision-making when surgery is required.

OBSTETRIC FACTORS IN PREGNANT WOMEN WITH CROHN'S DISEASE

Women with well-controlled CD can expect to undergo a healthy pregnancy and vaginal delivery of a healthy baby with similar risks to other pregnant women. However, those with active CD should be considered at increased risk—both during pregnancy and with respect to mode of delivery.

Risk of vaginal tears

There is no increase in vaginal tears in most women with CD undergoing vaginal delivery[21] and therefore vaginal delivery should be offered where possible unless there are obstetric complications. However, women with active perianal CF may have an increased risk of perineal tears when undergoing vaginal delivery and therefore planned cesarean section (CS) should be considered.[22]

Role of episiotomy

The role of episiotomy in pregnant women with CD is controversial as very few studies have analyzed CD patients separately from those with other forms of IBD. A Cochrane review[23] has recommended that episiotomy should only be performed for obstetric indications and not as routine practice in women with CD. There are several small studies, which indicate that there is a higher rate of subsequent fistula formation or development of perianal CD in those who have undergone episiotomy.[24,25]

Risk of fecal incontinence

Although there is good evidence for the link between vaginal tears and subsequent impairment of fecal continence,[26] most large studies do not specifically report on outcomes in women with CD. There does not appear to be any link between vaginal delivery per se and fecal incontinence in women with IBD in most studies[27,28] but one smaller study did suggest such a link.[29] Overall, it is likely that the majority of women with CD and healthy pregnancies should be able to deliver vaginally with no increased risk of fecal incontinence compared to other women.

Cesarean section

Although the majority of women with CD can deliver vaginally there is a higher rate of cesarean section (CS) for pregnant women with CD, than for unaffected pregnant women. CD patients are more likely to receive care from an obstetrician directly and therefore are more likely to be offered interventions. A study of approximately 4.2 million deliveries in USA showed a higher rate of CS for women with CD than for those without (45.9% vs 30.9%). Within the CD subgroup, those with perianal CD were more likely to undergo a CS than those with luminal CD only (83.1% vs 42.5%).[30]

Factors, which increase the risk of undergoing CS for pregnant women with CD include active perianal disease, fetal growth abnormalities, and maternal ill health. This is complicated further by healthcare systems across the world, which either encourage or discourage interventional delivery.

There is also some evidence that perianal CD may worsen in the 1st year postpartum[19,31] even if they undergo CS.[32] There is no evidence that CS is protective against the development of perianal CD.

There is an increased risk of complications after CS in women with CD and therefore vaginal delivery is recommended, whenever possible.[15] Those most at risk of complications are women who have an active flare of CD at the time of the delivery. This emphasizes the importance of managing pregnant women to achieve optimum control of CD prior to, and during pregnancy.

> **Key points for clinical practice**
> - Women with CD have an overall lower rate of fecundity than healthy women.
> - A collaborative multidisciplinary approach between gastroenterologists, surgeons, and obstetricians is important to manage pregnancy and delivery issues in women with CD.
> - Disease control of the mother preconception is likely to ensure the best outcome for the baby.
> - Knowledge of those CD-related medications which are teratogenic or otherwise contraindicated during pregnancy is essential.
> - Most pregnant women with CD can undergo vaginal delivery with satisfactory outcomes.
> - However, there is a higher rate of CS in pregnant women with CD, particularly those with perianal CD.
> - Women with CD should be offered CS for the same indications as other women.
> - Women with active perianal CD should consider elective CS.

REFERENCES

1. Haubich WS. Crohn of Crohn's disease. Gastroenterology. 1999;116:1034.
2. Campos FG, Kotze PG. Burrill Bernard Crohn (1884-1983): the man behind the disease. ABCD Arq Bras Cir Dig. 2013;26(4):253-5.
3. Aufses AH. The History of Crohn's Disease. Surg Clin North Am. 2001;81(1):1-11.
4. Cornish J, Tan E, Teare J, et al. A meta-analysis on the influence of inflammatory bowel disease on pregnancy. Gut. 2007;56(6):830-7.
5. IBD standards group. (2009). Quality Care Service Standards for the people who have inflammatory bowel disease (IBD). British Society of Gastroenterology. [online] Available from http://www.bsg.org.uk/attachments/160_IBDstandards.pdf. [Accessed September, 2017].
6. Selinger CP, Eaden J, Warwick S, et al. Inflammatory Bowel Disease and Pregnancy: Lack of knowledge is associated with negative views. J Crohns Colitis. 2013;7(6):e206-13.
7. Woude CJ, Ardizzone S, Bengtson MB, et al. The second European evidenced-based consensus on reproduction and pregnancy in inflammatory bowel disease. J Crohns Colitis. 2015;9(2):1-18.
8. Castiglione F, Pignata S, Morace F, et al. Effect of pregnancy on the clinical course of a cohort of women with inflammatory bowel disease. Ital J Gastroenterol. 1996;28(4):199-204.
9. Nørgård B, Hundborg HH, Jacobsen BA, et al. Disease activity in pregnant women with Crohn's disease and birth outcomes: a regional Danish cohort study. Am J Gastroenterol. 2007;102(9):1947-54.
10. Park-Wylie JD. Birth defects after maternal exposure to corticosteroids: prospective cohort study and meta-analysis of epidemiological studies. Teratology. 2000;62(6):385-92.

11. Beaulieu DB, Ananthakrishnan AN, Issa M, et al. Budesonide induction and maintenance therapy for Crohn's disease during pregnancy. Inflamm Bowel Dis. 2009;15(1):25-8.
12. Diav-Citrin O, Park YH, Veerasuntharam G, et al. The safety of mesalamine in human pregnancy: a prospective controlled cohort study. Gastroenterology. 1998;114(1):23-8.
13. Mahadevan U, Kane S, Sandborn WJ. Intentional infliximab use during pregnancy for induction or maintenance of remission of Crohn's disease. Aliment Pharmacol Ther. 2005;21(6):733-8.
14. Johnson DL, Jones KL, Chambers CD, et al. Pregnancy outcomes in women exposed to adalimumab: the OTIS autoimmune diseases in pregnancy project. Gastroenterology. 2009;136(5):A-27.
15. Richter JE. Gastroesophageal reflux disease during pregnancy. Gastroenterol Clin North Am. 2003;32(1):235-61.
16. Nikfar S, Abdollahi M, Moretti ME, et al. Use of proton-pump inhibitors during pregnancy and rates of major malformations: a meta-analysis. Dig Dis Sci. 2002;47(7):1526-9.
17. Soliman F, Hargest R. Intestinal failure in gastrointestinal fistula patients. Surgery. 2015;33(5):220-5.
18. Hyder SA, Travis SP, Jewell DP, et al. Fistulating anal Crohn's disease: results of combined surgical and infliximab treatment. Dis Colon Rectum. 2006;49(12):1837-41.
19. Topstad DR, Panaccione R, Heine JA, et al. Combined seton placement, infliximab infusion, and maintenance immunosuppressives improving healing rate in fistulising anorectal Crohn's disease. A single center experience. Dis Colon Rectum. 2003;46(5):577-83.
20. Van der Hagen SJ, Baeten CG, Soeters PB, et al. Anti-TNF-alpha (infliximab) used as induction treatment in case of active proctitis in a multistep strategy followed by definitive surgery of complex anal fistulas in Crohn's disease: a preliminary report. Dis Colon Rectum. 2005;48(4):758-67.
21. Broms G, Granath F, Linder M, et al. Complications from inflammatory bowel disease during pregnancy and delivery. Clin Gastroenterol Hepatol. 2012;10(11):1246-52.
22. Hatch Q, Champagne BJ, Maykel JA, et al. Crohn's disease and pregnancy: the impact of perianal disease on delivery methods and complications. Dis Colon Rectum. 2014;57(2):174-8.
23. Caroli G, Mignini L. Episiotomy for vaginal birth. Cochrane Database Syst Rev. 2009;1:CD000081.
24. Coremans G, Baert P, Rutgeerts J, et al. Episiotomy, a cause of ano-vaginal fistula in patients with Crohn's disease. Gastroenterology. 1995;108(4):A4802.
25. Smink M, Lotgering FK, Albers L, et al. Effect of childbirth on the course of Crohn's disease: results from a retrospective Cohort Study in the Netherlands. BMC Gastroenterol. 2011;11:6.
26. Sultan AH, Kamm MA, Hudson CN, et al. Third degree obstetric anal sphincter tears: risk factors and outcome of primary repair. Br Med J. 1994;308(6933):887-91.
27. Norton C, Dibley LB, Bassett P. Faecal incontinence in inflammatory bowel disease: associations and effect on quality of life. J Crohns Colitis. 2013;7(8):e302-311.
28. Kanis SL, van Der WJ, Christien J. Vaginal delivery is not associated with fecal incontinence in IBD women. Gastroenterology. 2015;148:S784.
29. Ong JPL, Edwards GJ, Allison MC. Mode of delivery and risk of faecal incontinence in women with or without inflammatory bowel disease: questionnaire survey. Inflamm Bowel Dis. 2007;13(11):1391-4.
30. Nguyen GC, Boudreau H, Harris ML, et al. Outcomes of Obstetric Hospitalizations among Women with Inflammatory Bowel Disease in the United States. Clin Gastroenterol Hepatol. 2009;7(3):329-34.
31. Ilnyckyj A, Blanchard JF, Rawsthorne P, et al. Perianal Crohn's disease and pregnancy: role of the mode of delivery. Am J Gastroenterol. 1999,94(11):3274-8.
32. Rogers RG, Katz VL. Course of Crohn's disease during pregnancy and its effect on pregnancy outcome: a retrospective review. Am J Perinatol. 1995;12(4):262-4.

Section 7

Hepatobiliary Surgery

CHAPTER

11. Pyogenic Liver Abscess

Chapter 11

Pyogenic liver abscess

Benjamin JH Lee, K Sim, Vishal G Shelat

INTRODUCTION

Liver abscess is defined as a localized collection of suppurative material encapsulated within the liver parenchyma due to inflammatory necrosis secondary to bacterial, amoebic, or fungal pathogens.[1,2] A pyogenic liver abscess (PLA) due to bacterial infection is the most common. In the early 20th century, PLA occurred mostly in young males due to pylephlebitis secondary to appendicitis and had a high mortality (77%) **(Table 11.1)**.[3] In the late 20th century, benign and malignant biliary tract disease emerged as leading causes.[2,4-7] More recently, invasive hepatobiliary interventions such as radiofrequency ablation (RFA), transarterial chemoembolization (TACE), and liver transplants have emerged as important etiologies.[8-11]

The incidence of PLA differs widely[12] and accounts for approximately 48% of all visceral abscesses.[13] Population studies report an incidence from 1.1 to 3.6 per 100,000 in the West and up to 17.6 per 100,000 in Asia.[13-17] PLA incidence is higher among males and increases with age.[2,14-15] With advances in interventional radiology, critical care, and a shift from surgical to a nonoperative management strategy, outcomes have improved. Nevertheless, mortality remains high.[18,19]

Table 11.1: Case series reporting on more than 300 patients with pyogenic liver abscess.

Author (reference)	Country	Study period	Population	Age (mean/median)	Predominant bacteria	Mortality (%)
Meddings L et al.[19]	USA	1994–2005	17,787	NR	Streptococcus	5.6
Keller JJ et al.[1]	Taiwan	2006–2008	12,050	62	KP	NR
Tsai FC et al.[16]	Taiwan	1996–2004	30,209	61	KP	10.9
Jepsen P et al.[15]	Denmark	1977–2002	1,448	64.2	NR	19.0
Lo JZ et al.[18]	Singapore	1994–2007	741	62	KP	14.0
Foo NP et al.[20]	Taiwan	2001–2004	377	60.1	KP	NR
Jun CH et al.[21]	China	2004–2013	602	62.6	KP	4.3
Chen SC et al.[22]	Taiwan	1999–2007	560	56.4	KP	9.1
Tian LT et al.[23]	China	2005–2009	357	60.1	KP	7.0
Chou FF et al.[24]	Taiwan	1986–1995	483	55.3	KP	15.5

(KP: *Klebsiella pneumoniae*; USA: United States of America; NR: Not reported).

RISK FACTORS

Risk factors predisposing to PLA include male gender,[3,6,7] advanced age,[23] diabetes mellitus (DM),[4,23,25] liver cirrhosis,[26] proton-pump inhibitor use,[27] and compromised immune function.[28] DM has a high prevalence and hence is commonly reported.[23] Impaired immune function in DM increases the risk of multiple abscesses[24] and *Klebsiella pneumoniae* infection.[3] Risk factors associated with increased mortality include male gender,[16,19] advanced age,[1,29] bacteremia, hyperbilirubinemia,[17,24] liver cirrhosis,[17,24] renal failure,[17,24] the presence of septic shock,[17,24,30] an APACHE (acute physiology and chronic health evaluation) II score of more than or equal to 15,[7] underlying malignancy,[1,16,19] and the presence of gas-forming PLA (GFPLA).[21] GFPLA, liver cirrhosis, size more than or equal to 6 cm and DM are associated with spontaneous rupture.[6,31,32]

CLASSIFICATION OF PYOGENIC LIVER ABSCESS

Pyogenic liver abscess can be classified based on etiology, bacteriology, and radiological features.

Etiology

Pyogenic liver abscesses can be primary or secondary. Primary etiologies involve direct seeding of pathogens following biliary, colonic, appendix related, hematogenous, or cryptogenic sepsis. Infection through the hepatobiliary tree remains the most common primary infection (30–50%). However, recent evidence suggests that it may be decreasing.[33] Infection arises from biliary stasis leading to elevated intrabiliary pressures, cholangiovenous reflux, and endotoxemia. This occurs in the setting of choledocholithiasis, biliary stricture, obstructive lesions, or congenital biliary tract abnormalities.[2,7,34]

Seeding of the portal venous system has been reported to be the second most common etiology in the setting of intra-abdominal infections. This contributes up to 20% of all cases.[2,35,36] The mechanism of infection involves a breach of the bowel mucosa leading to pylephlebitis.[5,7] Less commonly, hematogenous seeding can occur as a consequence of systemic bacteremia from either secondary causes of infection (endocarditis and pyelonephritis), intravenous (IV) drug abuse, or traumatic and vascular injury.[35,37] **Figure 11.1** shows a computerized tomography (CT) scan image of a patient with fish bone perforation of the distal stomach with contiguous PLA. Cryptogenic PLA is diagnosed when an exhaustive workup fails to establish the etiology. Malignancy needs to be excluded in patients with cryptogenic PLA.

Secondary etiologies involve complications of an underlying pathology or intervention. In giant tumors, areas of central necrosis can predispose to seeding. Therapeutic interventions such as RFA and TACE procedures induce areas of necrosis that act as a nidus for infection.[8-10,38] **Figure 11.2** shows a CT scan of a patient with hepatocellular carcinoma (HCC) treated with TACE who developed PLA secondary to infection in the necrotic tumor. We routinely prescribe prophylactic antibiotics in patients scheduled for RFA or TACE. PLA as a complication of biliary procedures including endobiliary stenting and sphincterotomy is common[35] as shown in **Figure 11.3**. **Figure 11.4** shows a dye study of the same patient after percutaneous drainage (PD). The contrast flows from the abscess cavity into the biliary ducts. Hepatobiliary surgical procedures can also predispose to PLA.[14] **Figure 11.5** shows PLA in a patient following a Whipple's procedure—the inset demonstrates aerobilia from a patent bilioenteric anastomosis.

Classification of pyogenic liver abscess

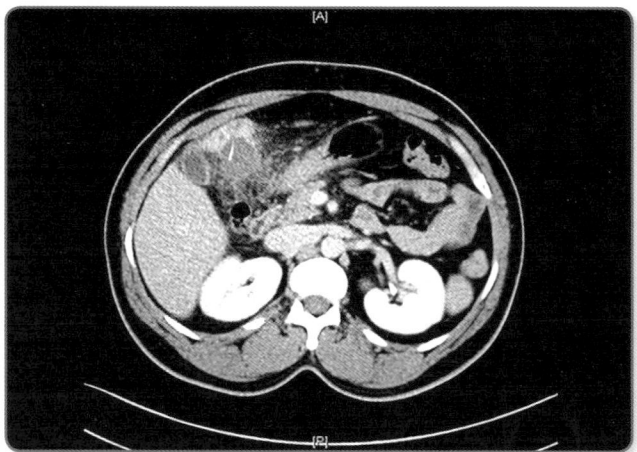

Figure 11.1 Pyogenic liver abscess (PLA) arising from foreign body perforation of gastric antrum.

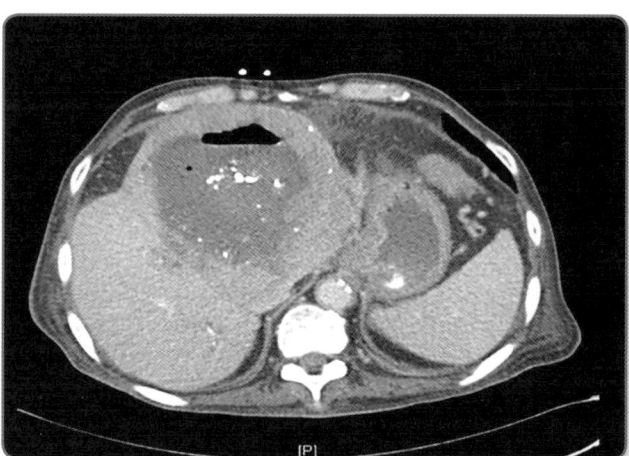

Figure 11.2 Pyogenic liver abscess (PLA) in patient following multiple transarterial chemoembolization (TACE).

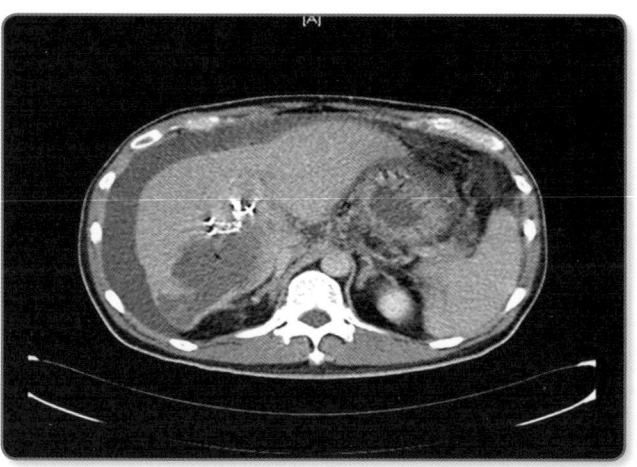

Figure 11.3 Pyogenic liver abscess (PLA) in patient following endobiliary stenting.

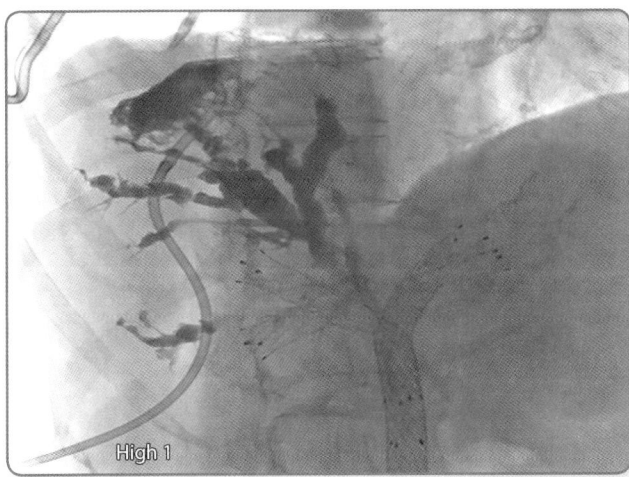

Figure 11.4 Pyogenic liver abscess (PLA) drainage tube study cholangiogram showing communication with segment 8 ducts.

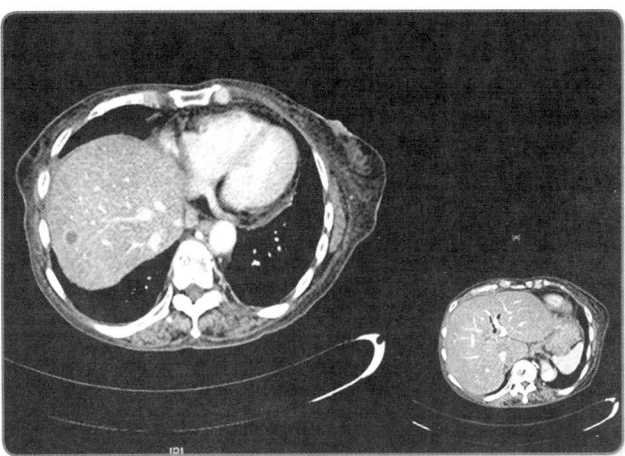

Figure 11.5 Pyogenic liver abscess (PLA) in patient 6 months post-hepaticojejunostomy following a Whipple's procedure—(inset) aerobilia from bilioenteric anastomosis.

Bacteriology

Pyogenic liver abscess may be monomicrobial or polymicrobial. Polymicrobial PLAs are common and involve mixed enteric facultative and anaerobic species.[13] *Klebsiella pneumoniae* has emerged as a leading pathogen of monomicrobial PLA.[39,40] Monomicrobial *Klebsiella pneumoniae* may be associated with colorectal cancer[41-43] and *Clostridium perfringens* is associated with high mortality.[44]

In 15–80% of cases, no organisms are detected. Reasons for failure of identification include the absence of routine use of advanced microbial detection techniques, noncompliance with institutional sepsis guidelines and avoidance of aspiration or drainage in a clinically improving patient.[43-46] Recently, we have reported the importance of recognizing such culture-negative PLA (CNPLA) and demonstrated that empiric treatment of CNPLA based on a local protocol is safe.[47]

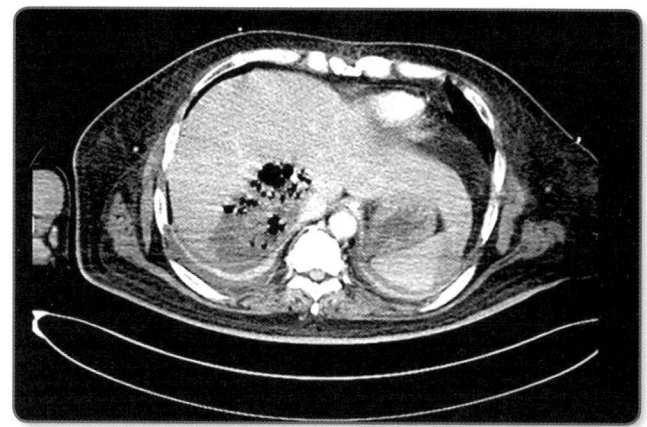

Figure 11.6 Gas-forming pyogenic liver abscess (GFPLA).

Radiological features

Most PLA are solitary and affect the right hemiliver. The size and number of abscesses are important determinants of management and outcomes. PLA can be classified based on size as small (≤4 cm), large (>4 and <10 cm), or giant (≥10 cm), and by number as either solitary or multiple. In general, small multiple abscesses are treated with antimicrobial therapy and large solitary abscesses require additional percutaneous needle aspiration or catheter drainage.[48] Giant abscesses may require surgical drainage. A small number of patients with PLA have radiological evidence of gas formation. **Figure 11.6** shows the CT scan of a patient with a large primary cryptogenic GFPLA. The incidence of GFPLA ranges from 5.6% to 31.8% and they are often cryptogenic. GFPLA is associated with diabetes mellitus and carries a high mortality (44.4%).[49]

DIAGNOSIS

Symptoms and signs

The clinical presentation of PLA is nonspecific, and hence a high index of suspicion is required.[50] Common symptoms include right upper abdominal pain, malaise, chills, pyrexia, nausea and vomiting, jaundice, anorexia, and weight loss.[2,3,50,51] Patients may demonstrate clinical signs specific to etiology, e.g. Murphy's sign.[43,51] Patients may reveal signs of systemic bacteremia including hypotension, respiratory distress, and altered mental state. Traditionally, the classic presentation of PLA is a triad of fever, right upper abdominal pain, and jaundice, but it is now seldom seen.[46]

INVESTIGATIONS

Biochemical

Laboratory findings in patients with PLA are nonspecific. Elevated C-reactive protein (CRP), erythrocyte sedimentation rate (ESR), white blood cell count, and procalcitonin are sensitive but not specific to PLA. Serum alkaline phosphatase (ALP) is elevated in up to 90% of patients and suggests biliary etiology. Deranged liver enzymes, serum creatinine more than 100 μmol/L, urea more than 8.1 mmol/L, international normalized ratio (INR) more than 1.5, albumin less than 3 g/L, and hemoglobin less than 100 g/L are also seen.[2,19,22,52,53] CRP levels may independently determine duration of antibiotic therapy.[54] Abnormalities in biomarkers often prompt imaging studies that establish the diagnosis and underlying etiology.

Imaging

Ultrasonography (USG) and CT scan of the abdomen and pelvis are both sensitive for establishing diagnosis of PLA.[50] On USG, PLA is poorly demarcated and may vary from hyperechoic to hypoechoic.[55] GFPLA have characteristically high echogenicity.[56] Color Doppler USG demonstrates an absence of central perfusion in PLA, differentiating it from focal benign and malignant lesions. Contrast-enhanced USG shows marginal wall enhancement in the arterial phase and progressive venous hypoenhancement in the portal and late phases. The lack of enhancement in liquefied necrotic areas is the most prominent feature of PLA.[54,55] USG scan is the modality of choice for monitoring the response to treatment and establish resolution. In our institution, CT scan is the first-line investigation for acute abdomen, as it is available after office hours and avoids a potential delay in diagnosis and management. CT scan establishes the diagnosis of PLA and provides details regarding location, size, internal loculations, and primary abdominal pathology. On CT scan, PLA has peripheral rim enhancement and central attenuation.[57] PLA can appear solid, contain gas or air fluid levels, and exhibit circumferential perfusion abnormalities.[57] In patients with normal gallbladder on CT scan, USG scan of abdomen is routinely performed to rule out gallstones. Magnetic resonance imaging (MRI) shows central hypointensity on T1-weighted imaging and hyperintense signals on T2-weighted imaging.[58,59] Diffusion-weighted imaging (DWI) MRI tends to exhibit high-signal intensity within PLA.[60]

PRINCIPLES OF TREATMENT

Nonoperative management

Antibiotics

Intravenous antibiotics are essential first-line management in patients with sepsis.[61] Small solitary or multiple (≤4 cm) primary PLA can usually be treated solely with antibiotics. Secondary PLA will need source control measures. Combination therapy with percutaneous aspiration or catheter drainage is indicated when PLA is large and accessible.[62] Switching from IV to oral formulations and duration of treatment are decided according to local protocols and treatment response. In a local study involving 288 patients, the median duration of IV antibiotic treatment was 14 days, and 62% of patients required PD in addition to antibiotics.[63]

Percutaneous drainage

Needle aspiration is reserved for solitary uniloculated PLA.[64-66] PD provides better response rates and allows prompt resolution of PLA compared to needle aspiration alone.[67] Needle aspiration, however, has advantages of being a simple procedure that causes less discomfort.[68] The mathematical principles regarding the volume of a sphere reveal that PLA of 3, 4, and 5 cm diameter will have an estimated volume of 14 cc, 34 cc, and 65 cc, respectively. We propose that a large abscess should have PD in preference to needle aspiration. PD is generally preferred over surgical drainage, as it avoids risks associated with surgery and anesthesia. PD has a high-success rate in unilocular solitary PLA. PD has risks of drainage site skin sepsis, tube blockage, and tube dislodgement.[62] In patients with multiloculated PLA, multiple drains may be required to control sepsis.

Surgery

Surgical drainage is reserved for patients with predicted risk of PD failure or who have already failed nonoperative management. We define failure of nonoperative management as having signs of sepsis after 5 days of IV antibiotics and PD.[63] Surgical drainage is usually preferred for giant PLA.[68] Evidence is available suggesting that rates of successful treatment with surgical drainage are higher compared to PD for giant PLA, though morbidity rates are comparable.[69] Other factors favoring surgical drainage include multiloculated or high-viscosity abscesses, having an underlying surgical condition requiring surgery and a short length to liver capsule (<0.25 cm).[68] Multiloculated or giant PLAs are not ideal for PD. However, these are not absolute contraindications and we have reported that PD is safe and sufficient even in giant PLA.[70] Laparoscopic drainage is less invasive and remains an option in units with appropriate technical expertise.[71] Video-assisted surgical drainage is an option in patients with persistent PLA following PD.[62] This is akin to the "step-up" approach for pancreatic necrosectomy. Video-assisted drainage is safe, feasible, and has low morbidity.[62] However, more data is required before the "step-up" approach is widely adopted in routine clinical practice. In our experience, PD is safe and sufficient even for giant PLA and hence the role of operative strategies is limited. The only absolute indication for surgical drainage is a necessity to operate for primary pathology responsible for the PLA or in patients with ruptured PLA.

PROGNOSIS

Free intraperitoneal rupture and invasion to neighboring organs are risks of PLA.[72] Risk factors for rupture include size more than 6 cm, liver cirrhosis, and the presence of gas.[21] Emergency surgery is indicated for free rupture, while antimicrobial therapy with PD can be considered for localized rupture to neighboring organs.[21] Invasive liver abscess syndrome can result in both intrahepatic and extrahepatic symptoms. *Klebsiella pneumoniae* is emerging as an important cause of endophthalmitis.[73] The morbidity of PLA is high in the elderly and diabetics.[45] Other important causes of mortality include multiorgan failure, pneumonia, sepsis, and hepatocellular carcinoma.[63]

> **Key points for clinical practice**
> - Pyogenic liver abscess is the most common visceral abscess.
> - Male gender and advanced age are important risk factors for PLA and associated with mortality risk.
> - Widespread application of RFA and TACE procedures for liver malignancy is associated with increasing incidence of PLA.
> - The majority of PLA is polymicrobial. Culture-negative PLA is common in routine clinical practice.

- Imaging is essential to establish a diagnosis of PLA and guide treatment.
- Antibiotics and PD are cornerstones of PLA treatment. Surgical drainage is reserved for patients with failure of nonoperative treatment or intraperitoneal rupture.
- Giant PLA may require surgical drainage. Gas-forming PLA is associated with high mortality.

REFERENCES

1. Keller JJ, Tsai MC, Lin CC, et al. Risk of infections subsequent to pyogenic liver abscess: a nationwide population-based study. Clin Microbiol Infect. 2013;19(8):717-22.
2. Huang CJ, Pitt HA, Lipsett PA, et al. Pyogenic hepatic abscess. Changing trends over 42 years. Ann Surg. 1996;223(5):600-9.
3. Ochsner A, DeBakey M, Murray S. Pyogenic abscess of the liver. Am J Surg. 1938;40(1):292-353.
4. Lee KT, Wong SR, Sheen PC. Pyogenic liver abscess: an audit of 10 years' experience and analysis of risk factors. Dig Surg. 2001;18(6):459-65; discussion 465-6.
5. Kumar D, Ramanathan S, Al Faki A, et al. Faecolith migrating from the appendix to produce liver abscess after subhepatic laparoscopic appendectomy. Trop Doct. 2015;45(5):241-4.
6. Law ST, Li KK. Is hepatic neoplasm-related pyogenic liver abscess a distinct clinical entity? World J Gastroenterol. 2012;18(10):1110-6.
7. Murarka S, Pranav F, Dandavate V. Pyogenic liver abscess secondary to disseminated streptococcus anginosus from sigmoid diverticulitis. J Glob Infect Dis. 2011;3(1):79-81.
8. Huang SF, Ko CW, Chang CS, et al. Liver abscess formation after transarterial chemoembolization for malignant hepatic tumor. Hepatogastroenterology. 2003;50(52):1115-8.
9. Iida H, Aihara T, Ikuta S, et al. Risk of abscess formation after liver tumour radiofrequency ablation: A review of 8 cases with a history of enterobiliary anastomosis. Hepatogastroenterology. 2014;61(135):1867-70.
10. Elias D, Di Pietroantonio D, Gachot B, et al. Liver abscess after radiofrequency ablation of tumors in patients with a biliary tract procedure. Gastroenterol Clin Biol. 2006;30(6-7):823-7.
11. Hoffmann R, Rempp H, Schmidt D, et al. Prolonged antibiotic prophylaxis in patients with bilioenteric anastomosis undergoing percutaneous radiofrequency ablation. J Vasc Interv Radiol. 2012;23(4):545-51.
12. Lin YT, Liu CJ, Chen TJ, et al. Pyogenic liver abscess as the initial manifestation of underlying hepatocellular carcinoma. Am J Med. 2011;124(12):1158-64.
13. Altemeier WA, Culbertson WR, Fullen WD, et al. Intra-abdominal abscesses. Am J Surg. 1973;125(1):70.
14. Kaplan GG, Gregson DB, Laupland KB. Population-based study of the epidemiology of and the risk factors for pyogenic liver abscess. Clin Gastroenterol Hepatol. 2004;2(11):1032-8.
15. Jepsen P, Vilstrup H, Schønheyder HC, et al. A nationwide study of the incidence and 30-day mortality rate of pyogenic liver abscess in Denmark, 1977-2002. Aliment Pharmacol Ther. 2005;21(10):1185-8.
16. Tsai FC, Huang YT, Chang LY, et al. Pyogenic Liver Abscess as Endemic Disease, Taiwan. Emerg Infect Dis. 2008;14(10):1592-600.
17. Mohsen AH, Green ST, Read RC, et al. Liver abscess in adults: ten years experience in a UK centre. QJM. 2002;95(12):797-802.
18. Lo JZW, Leow JJ, Ng PLF, et al. Predictors of therapy failure in a series of 741 adult pyogenic liver abscesses. J Hepatobiliary Pancreat Sci. 2015;22(2):156-65.
19. Meddings L, Myers RP, Hubbard J, et al. A population-based study of pyogenic liver abscesses in the United States: incidence, mortality, and temporal trends. Am J Gastroenterol. 2010;105(1):117-24.
20. Foo NP, Chen KT, Lin HJ, et al. Characteristics of pyogenic liver abscess patients with and without diabetes mellitus. Am J Gastroenterol. 2010;105(2):328-35.
21. Jun CH, Yoon JH, Wi JW, et al. Risk factors and clinical outcomes for spontaneous rupture of pyogenic liver abscess. J Dig Dis. 2015;16(1):31-6.
22. Chen SC, Lee YT, Yen CH, et al. Pyogenic liver abscess in the elderly: clinical features, outcomes and prognostic factors. Age Ageing. 2009;38(3):271-6.
23. Tian LT, Yao K, Zhang XY, et al. Liver abscesses in adult patients with and without diabetes mellitus: an analysis of the clinical characteristics, features of the causative pathogens, outcomes and predictors of fatality: a report based on a large population, retrospective study in China. Clin Microbiol Infect. 2012;18(9):E314-30.
24. Alvarez Pérez JA, González JJ, Baldonedo RF, et al. Clinical course, treatment, and multivariate analysis of risk factors for pyogenic liver abscess. Am J Surg. 2001;181(2):177-86.

25. Jeong SW, Jang JY, Lee TH, et al. Cryptogenic pyogenic liver abscess as the herald of colon cancer. J Gastroenterol Hepatol. 2012;27(2):248-55.
26. Mølle I, Thulstrup AM, Vilstrup H, et al. Increased risk and case fatality rate of pyogenic liver abscess in patients with liver cirrhosis: a nationwide study in Denmark. Gut. 2001;48(2):260-3.
27. Wang YP, Liu CJ, Chen TJ, et al. Proton pump inhibitor use significantly increases the risk of cryptogenic liver abscess: a population-based study. Aliment Pharmacol Ther. 2015;41(11):1175-81.
28. Morii K, Kashihara A, Miura S, et al. Successful hepatectomy for intraperitoneal rupture of pyogenic liver abscess caused by Klebsiella pneumoniae. Clin J Gastroenterol. 2012;5(2):136-40.
29. Law ST, Li KK. Older age as a poor prognostic sign in patients with pyogenic liver abscess. Int J Infect Dis. 2013;17(3):e177-84.
30. Ruiz-Hernández JJ, León-Mazorra M, Conde-Martel A, et al. Pyogenic liver abscesses: mortality-related factors. Eur J Gastroenterol Hepatol. 2007;19(10):853-8.
31. Liew KVS, Lau TC, Ho CH, et al. Pyogenic liver abscess—a tropical centre's experience in management with review of current literature. Singapore Med J. 2000;41(10):489-92.
32. Law ST, Kong Li MK. Is there any difference in pyogenic liver abscess caused by Streptococcus milleri and Klebsiella spp? retrospective analysis over a 10-year period in a regional hospital. J Microbiol Immunol Infect. 2013;46(1):11-8.
33. Eltawansy SA, Merchant C, Atluri P, et al. Multi-organ failure secondary to a Clostridium perfringens gaseous liver abscess following a self-limited episode of acute gastroenteritis. Am J Case Rep. 2015;16:182-6.
34. Kwan KEL, Shelat VG, Tan CH. Recurrent pyogenic cholangitis: a review of imaging findings and clinical management. Abdom Radiol (NY). 2017;42(1):46-56.
35. Wong WM, Wong BCY, Hui CK, et al. Pyogenic liver abscess: retrospective analysis of 80 cases over a 10-year period. J Gastroenterol Hepatol. 2002;17(9):1001-7.
36. McDonald MI. Pyogenic liver abscess: diagnosis, bacteriology and treatment. Eur J Clin Microbiol. 1984;3(6):506-9.
37. Seeto RK, Rockey DC. Pyogenic liver abscess. Changes in etiology, management, and outcome. Medicine (Baltimore). 1996;75(2):99-113.
38. Shin JU, Kim KM, Shin SW, et al. A prediction model for liver abscess developing after transarterial chemoembolization in patients with hepatocellular carcinoma. Dig Liver Dis. 2014;46(9):813-7.
39. Chen CH, Wu SS, Chang HC, et al. Initial presentations and final outcomes of primary pyogenic liver abscess: a cross-sectional study. BMC Gastroenterol. 2014;14:133.
40. Qu K, Liu C, Wang ZX, et al. Pyogenic liver abscesses associated with nonmetastatic colorectal cancers: an increasing problem in Eastern Asia. World J Gastroenterol. 2012;18(23):2948-55.
41. Kao WY, Hwang CY, Chang YT, et al. Cancer risk in patients with pyogenic liver abscess: a nationwide cohort study. Aliment Pharmacol Ther. 2012;36(5):467-76.
42. Huang WK, Chang JWC, See LC, et al. Higher rate of colorectal cancer among patients with pyogenic liver abscess with Klebsiella pneumoniae than those without: an 11-year follow-up study. Colorectal Dis. 2012;14(12):e794-801.
43. Lai HC, Lin CC, Cheng KS, et al. Increased incidence of gastrointestinal cancers among patients with pyogenic liver abscess: a population-based cohort study. Gastroenterology. 2014;146(1):129-37.e1.
44. Khan MS, Ishaq MK, Jones KR. Gas-Forming Pyogenic Liver Abscess with Septic Shock. Case Rep Crit Care. 2015;2015:632873.
45. Liao CH, Huang YT, Chang CY, et al. Capsular serotypes and multilocus sequence types of bacteremic Klebsiella pneumoniae isolates associated with different types of infections. Eur J Clin Microbiol Infect Dis. 2014;33(3):365-9.
46. Berg GM, Vasquez DG, Hale LS, et al. Evaluation of process variations in noncompliance in the implementation of evidence-based sepsis care. J Health Qual. 2013;35(1):60-9.
47. Shelat VG, Wang Q, Chia CL, et al. Patients with culture negative pyogenic liver abscess have the same outcomes compared to those with Klebsiella pneumoniae pyogenic liver abscess. Hepatobiliary Pancreat Dis Int. 2016;15(5):504-11.
48. Klink C, Binnebösel M, Schmeding M, et al. Video-assisted hepatic abscess debridement. HPB (Oxford). 2015;17(8):732-5.
49. Chou FF, Sheen-Chen SM, Chen YS, et al. The comparison of clinical course and results of treatment between gas-forming and non-gas-forming pyogenic liver abscess. Arch Surg. 1995;130(4):401-5; discussion 406.
50. Lardière-Deguelte S, Ragot E, Amroun K, et al. Hepatic abscess: diagnosis and management. J Visc Surg. 2015;152(4):231-43.

51. Alkofer B, Dufay C, Parienti JJ, et al. Are pyogenic liver abscesses still a surgical concern? A Western experience. HPB Surg. 2012;2012:316013.
52. Longworth S, Han J. Pyogenic liver abscess. Clin Liver Disease. 2015;6:51-4.
53. Rahimian J, Wilson T, Oram V, et al. Pyogenic liver abscess: recent trends in etiology and mortality. Clin Infect Dis. 2004;39(11):1654-9.
54. Gao HN, Yuan WX, Yang MF, et al. Clinical significance of C-reactive protein values in antibiotic treatment for pyogenic liver abscess. World J Gastroenterol. 2010;16(38):4871-5.
55. Chen LD, Xu HX, Xie XY, et al. Intrahepatic cholangiocarcinoma and hepatocellular carcinoma: differential diagnosis with contrast-enhanced ultrasound. Eur Radiol. 2010;20(3):743-53.
56. Kuligowska E, Connors S, Shapiro J. Liver abscess: sonography in diagnosis and treatment. Am J Roentgenol. 1982;138(2):253-7.
57. Bächler P, Baladron MJ, Menias C, et al. Multimodality imaging of liver infections: differential diagnosis and potential pitfalls. Radiographics. 2016;36:1001-23.
58. Méndez RJ, Schiebler ML, Outwater EK, et al. Hepatic abscesses: MR imaging findings. Radiology. 1994;190(2):431-6.
59. Balci NC, Semelka RC, Noone TC, et al. Pyogenic hepatic abscesses: MRI findings on T1- and T2-weighted and serial gadolinium-enhanced gradient-echo images. J Magn Reson Imaging. 1999;9(2):285-90.
60. Chan JH, Tsui EY, Luk SH, et al. Diffusion-weighted MR imaging of the liver: distinguishing hepatic abscess from cystic or necrotic tumor. Abdom Imaging. 2001;26(2):161-5.
61. Sartelli M, Weber DG, Ruppé E, et al. Antimicrobials: a global alliance for optimizing their rational use in intra-abdominal infections (AGORA). World J Emerg Surg. 2016;11:33.
62. Klink C, Binnebösel M, Schmeding M, et al. Video-assisted hepatic abscess debridement. HPB. 2015;17(8):732-5.
63. Shelat VG, Chia C, Yeo C, et al. Pyogenic liver abscess: does escherichia coli cause more adverse outcomes than klebsiella pneumoniae? World J Surg. 2015;39(10):2535-42.
64. Zerem E, Hadzic A. Sonographically guided percutaneous catheter drainage versus needle aspiration in the management of pyogenic liver abscess. AJR. 2007;189(3):W138-42.
65. Ch Yu S, Hg Lo R, Kan PS, et al. Pyogenic liver abscess: treatment with needle aspiration. Clin Radiol. 1997;52(12):912-6.
66. Rajak CL, Gupta S, Jain S, et al. Percutaneous treatment of liver abscesses: needle aspiration versus catheter drainage. AJR Am J Roentgenol. 1998;170(4):1035-9.
67. Yu S, Ho S, Lau W, et al. Treatment of pyogenic liver abscess: prospective randomized comparison of catheter drainage and needle aspiration. Hepatology. 2004;39(4):932-8.
68. Heneghan HM, Healy NA, Martin ST, et al. Modern management of pyogenic hepatic abscess: a case series and review of the literature. BMC Res Notes. 2011;4:80.
69. Bertel CK, van Heerden JA, Sheedy PF. Treatment of pyogenic hepatic abscesses. Surgical vs percutaneous drainage. Arch Surg. 1986;121(5):554-8.
70. Ahmed S, Chia CLK, Junnarkar SP, et al. Percutaneous drainage for giant pyogenic liver abscess—is it safe and sufficient? Am J Surg. 2016;211(1):95-101.
71. Aydin C, Piskin T, Sumer F, et al. Laparoscopic drainage of pyogenic liver abscess. JSLS. 2010;14(3):418-20.
72. Khan NA, Choudhury S, Jhanwar P. Ruptured liver abscess in neonates: report of two cases. J Neonatal Surg. 2016;5(3):7-9.
73. Fang CT, Lai SY, Yi WC, et al. Klebsiella pneumoniae genotype K1: an emerging pathogen that causes septic ocular or central nervous system complications from pyogenic liver abscess. Clin Infect Dis. 2007;45(3):284-93.

Section 8

Vascular Surgery

CHAPTER

12. **Thoracic Outlet Syndrome**

Chapter 12

Thoracic outlet syndrome

Georgiana Samoila, Ian M Williams

INTRODUCTION

Thoracic outlet syndrome (TOS) describes a spectrum of disorders affecting the neurovascular structures passing from the neck and upper chest region into the upper arm. TOS encompasses three different clinical entities—(1) venous, (2) arterial, and (3) neurologic, with extrinsic compression of one or more of these structures as the common denominator.

The most common type of TOS is the neurological type, representing more than 95% of all cases, followed by venous (2%) and arterial TOS (1%).[1,2]

Randomized controlled trials (RCTs) are scarce, due to lack of consensus on diagnosis and management, as concluded by a recent Cochrane Collaboration review of treatment for TOS in 2014.[3] A very recent document in 2016 by the Society for Vascular Surgery called for more consistency in the use of definitions for diagnosis and agreement on standard management strategies for TOS, especially the neurogenic type.[4]

ANATOMY OF THE THORACIC OUTLET

Peet, in 1956, first used the term "thoracic outlet syndrome" to describe clinical disorders affecting the vascular and neurological structures within the area extending from the supraclavicular fossa to the axilla, including the region between the clavicle and the first rib.[5] Anatomically, this area is normally referred to as the thoracic inlet (thoracic outlet is the anatomic region bound by the 12th rib and diaphragm). However, the term initially proposed by Peet (1956)[5] has persisted and continues to be used today in this context, to describe the space above the first rib extending as high as the fifth cervical nerve and medially to the upper mediastinum, with the superior surface of the first rib forming the floor, and the clavicle and subclavius muscle forming the roof.[5,6] A sound understanding of the anatomy of the thoracic outlet is essential for management of patients with TOS.

The subclavian vein (SV) is the most anterior structure at the thoracic outlet and runs anteriorly to the scalenus anterior muscle, proceeding laterally over the first rib, and inferior to the clavicle **(Figure 12.1)**.

The subclavian artery lies behind the SV and anterior scalene muscle and inferior to the brachial plexus with the medial scalene muscle posteriorly. The scalenus anterior and medius muscles elevate the first rib and flex the neck laterally. As they elevate the upper ribs, they also act as accessory muscles of respiration, along with sternocleidomastoid.

The subclavius muscle is a small triangular structure, with its tendon originating from the first rib and its cartilage anterior to the costoclavicular ligament. Its fibers proceed superolaterally and insert on the inferior aspect of the clavicle. The subclavius muscle depresses the shoulder and draws the clavicle anteriorly.

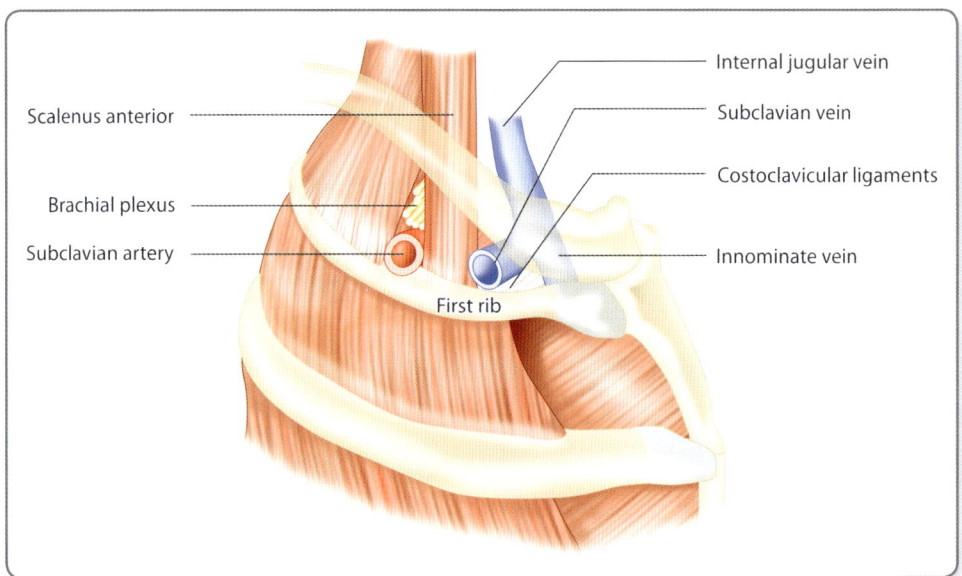

Figure 12.1 Normal thoracic outlet anatomy with subclavius muscle removed.

The subclavius muscle and tendon are located medially, which creates the potential for a nutcracker-like compression of the SV with very minimal movement. The costoclavicular ligament inserts inferiorly to the upper medial aspect of the cartilage of the first rib and proceeds posterolaterally to the costal tuberosity on the inferior aspect of the medial clavicle. Rigberg (2006)[6] described the "scissoring" effect between the clavicle and first rib with arm movement, to explain the potential for compression of neurovascular structures at the thoracic outlet.[6]

Compression causing TOS can occur at three different anatomic spaces—(1) the costoclavicular space (causing venous compression), (2) the interscalene triangle (arterial and nerve compression), and (3) pectoralis minor space (nerve compression).[4] Less commonly, the SV may be compressed at the pectoralis minor space.[4]

Cervical ribs

According to the Gruber classification, there are four categories of cervical rib.[7] Firstly, the cervical rib may be a complete rib, which articulates with the first rib or manubrium.[7] Secondly, it may be an incomplete rib and its anterior aspect may have a free end.[7] Thirdly, the anterior aspect of the incomplete rib may continue anteriorly with a fibrous band; and lastly, there may be just a short extra length of bone beyond the transverse process of the C7 vertebra.[7] Cervical ribs occur in 0.5-2% of the population and may cause compression of the brachial plexus and subclavian artery at the thoracic outlet (no association with venous TOS).[8]

First rib

The first rib usually lies flat in the horizontal plane in the shape of the letter "C". However, the rib may be anomalous and lie such that it resembles the letter "J" or may even be laterally placed with a broader mid section, which has the effect of an increased area over which vital structures pass. Other abnormalities comprise an incomplete floating first rib and even an articulation with the second rib directly instead of the manubrium.[9] The presence of an anomalous first rib may be harder to recognize as they originate from the transverse processes of the first thoracic vertebra. However, it is where they attach to distally and their orientation which may cause compression of neurovascular structures requiring surgical decompression.[10]

SURGICAL DECOMPRESSION OF THE THORACIC OUTLET

In 1861, Coote[11] described the thoracic outlet region as "*not a pleasant one for any procedure requiring the use of a knife*", after performing the first successful removal of a cervical rib in a patient with upper limb ischemia.[11] It appears that his statement is as true today as it was 155 years ago, since the potential for damage to important structures should not be underestimated. Structures that may be encountered during surgical decompression for TOS include the phrenic and dorsal scapular nerves, the thoracic duct and pleura surrounding the lung apex.

While historically, TOS has been considered one single entity, successful surgical decompression, and long-term durability should take into account its three distinct anatomic spaces.[12] The surgical approaches used for decompression are transaxillary (TA), supraclavicular, and infraclavicular (IC), with a further approach described using a paraclavicular (PC) incision.

NEUROLOGIC THORACIC OUTLET SYNDROME

Clinical presentation

Neurologic TOS (NTOS) represents approximately 97% of all cases of TOS and is caused by compression of the brachial plexus roots within the scalene triangle and/or the area under the pectoral space.[13] The condition predominantly affects women in their 30s. In many cases, there is a previous history of neck trauma. This may be relatively trivial, a more major injury or as a sequel to whiplash injuries. The relationship to the presence of a cervical rib is problematic, as most are asymptomatic. It is estimated that when a cervical rib is present only 1 in 20,000–80,000 of these individuals will be found to have true NTOS.[8]

Wilbourn (1988)[14] suggested the term "disputed" NTOS (also known as nonspecific NTOS) to describe cases of NTOS with "no generally accepted clinical or laboratory presentation", to distinguish this from "true" NTOS.[8,14] This distinction is important, as it appears that nonspecific TOS may be overdiagnosed; and more importantly, surgical treatment may not be as effective as in the case of "true" NTOS.

True neurogenic TOS is caused by compression of the lower trunks of the brachial plexus. A typical symptom is atrophy of the intrinsic muscles of the hand. Invariably, the lateral muscles of the hand are first affected. Patients are usually female with progressive symptoms and pain is frequent. Sensation is usually intact or minimally impaired.[15] Disputed neurogenic TOS is controversial, as the brachial plexus is compressed somewhere along its anatomic path. The most common locations are the interscalene triangle and between the first thoracic rib and other surrounding structures. Typically electromyography, which measures the muscular responses to nerve stimulation, is normal. Other tests include nerve conduction studies, which record the speed of impulses through a nerve—for disputed NTOS, these are invariably normal. One clinical feature is that pain associated with the condition which is worse with provocative movements.

Diagnosis

The diagnosis of neurological TOS can be difficult. Many tests have adopted upper limb and shoulder maneuvers, which may elicit symptoms. By placing the neck and arms in certain positions, this may place stress on the brachial plexus to produce symptoms of pain, numbness, and tingling in the hand, arm or neck. What is apparent is that these maneuvers can be misleading as positive responses are found in many healthy individuals. Other provocative tests provide better reliability and are seldom positive in healthy people. These include rotating the neck or tilting the head to one side causing symptoms to appear on the contralateral side.[1] The upper limb tension test is performed by extending one arm to the side, bending the wrist upward, and tilting the head to the opposite side.[1] When all of these maneuvers elicit the same symptoms, a diagnosis of neurologic TOS should be considered.

A helpful test is the scalene muscle block, which is performed by injecting a small amount of local anesthetic directly into the scalene muscles. A positive response is seen when there is an improvement in symptoms at rest as well as with the provocative maneuvers. A similar muscle block test is helpful in diagnosing neurogenic pectoralis minor syndrome. The scalene muscle block test had a positive predictive value for TOS of 90% in 122 patients studied by Jordan (1998),[16] with better outcomes following first rib resection in patients with a positive preoperative scalene block (94%) compared with those who had a negative scalene block (50%).[16]

Nerve tests such as electromyography and nerve conduction velocity tests are usually normal. Recent introduction of the medial antebrachial cutaneous nerve test has proven of use, particularly in people who have symptoms in just one arm.[1] The good arm serves as a baseline against which to compare the symptomatic arm. X-rays of the thoracic inlet are usually normal but may demonstrate an extra rib in the neck **(Figures 12.2A and B)**.

Differential diagnosis

In order to assess the need for decompression surgery at the thoracic outlet, it is important to exclude various conditions which may mimic NTOS. The differential diagnosis includes carpal tunnel syndrome, cervical disk disease, brachial plexus injuries, and rotator cuff injuries **(Table 12.1)**.

Conservative management

Nonsurgical treatment consists of physiotherapy to improve upper arm and shoulder mobility. Also important are posture exercises and reduction of scalene and pectoralis major spasms. The use of physiotherapy as the initial treatment is important and should be performed by someone with a particular interest in the condition as incorrect approaches may lead to unnecessary and prolonged treatment actions. The physiotherapy invariably lasts for many months before any long-term benefit is felt and hence active cooperation between patient and the physiotherapist is vital.

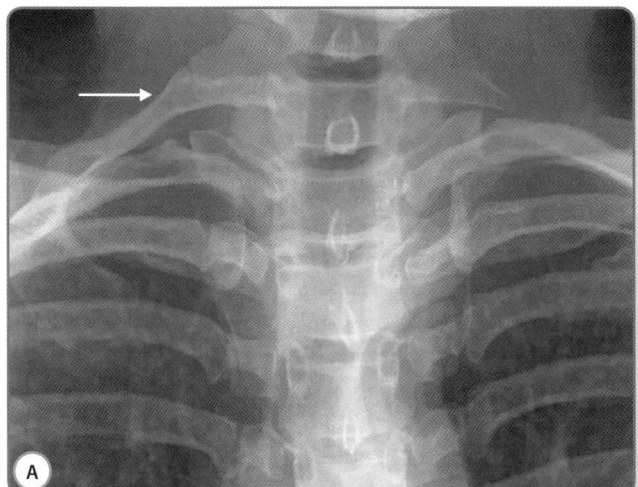
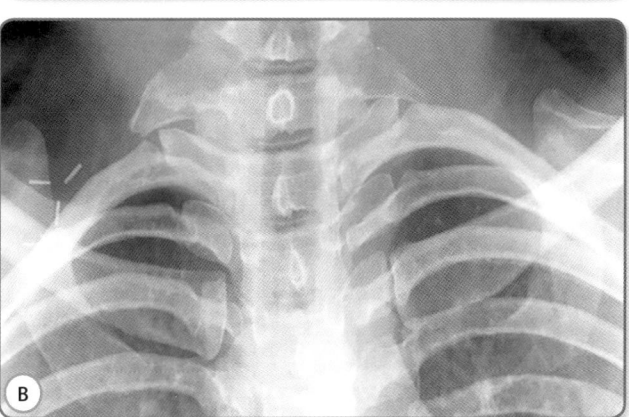

Figures 12.2A and B A 24-year-old female presenting with neurologic thoracic outlet syndrome (NTOS) of the right upper limb. (A) Thoracic spine X-ray—right cervical rib (arrow). (B) Postoperative imaging following removal of right cervical rib.

Table 12.1: Differential diagnosis of neurologic thoracic outlet syndrome (NTOS).[8]			
Clinical symptom/sign	NTOS	Late carpal tunnel syndrome	C8 or T1 radiculopathy
Pain	Prolonged history of pain on medial aspect of upper limb	Late feature	Neck pain elicited by neck movement, radiating into upper limb
Paresthesia	Uncommon	Intermittent symptoms at rest and with elevation	Accompanies pain radiating from neck into upper limb
Loss of sensation	Lower plexus distribution: Loss of sensation < weakness	Median nerve distribution (index and middle fingers)	Dermatomal distribution: Loss of sensation > weakness
Weakness	T1 > C8	Muscles innervated by median nerve distal to wrist	Myotomal distribution
Muscular atrophy	Thenar eminence (severe) Medial and distal forearm (less obvious)	Thenar eminence (moderate to severe)	Myotomal distribution (more apparent distally)

Surgical management

There is controversy, as to which patients with NTOS benefit from surgery. For those with true NTOS and symptoms and signs such as wasting of the intrinsic hand muscles, surgery should be considered for decompression. These patients have long-standing extrinsic compression of the neurovascular structures in the neck. Surgery for NTOS is performed to remove extrinsic compression of the nerve roots trunks or branches themselves. Structures which may need to be removed or modified in order to reduce compression are the scalene muscles, a first or a cervical rib if present or a fibrous band or scar tissue which may occur within the brachial plexus roots and trunks. Less commonly, compression of the brachial plexus posterior to the pectoralis minor tendon may cause NTOS.

Obtaining consent by full explanation of the proposed surgery is vital as a permanent cure cannot be guaranteed and there is the possibility of significant complications. Common complications include neurological, arterial and venous injury, pneumothorax, and damage to the long-thoracic nerve (LTN). The thoracic duct and its branches on the left side should be avoided. The two most common surgical approaches for NTOS are the TA and supraclavicular. For the supraclavicular surgery approach, a transverse skin incision is made a finger breadth above the clavicle. Once the skin is incised, the scalene fat pad is encountered and this is mobilized on its lateral pedicle away from the underlying tissue. The inferior belly of omohyoid is encountered and this can be incised with no problems. The scalenus anterior is then visualized and the principal structure to avoid here is the phrenic nerve, which runs from lateral to medial along its anterior surface. This is a fragile nerve, which needs to be handled very carefully. A sling can be applied to mobilize it and apply slight traction medially but even gentle manipulation may result in a palsy. The use of electrocautery for hemostasis is mandatory in this area due to proximity of neural tissue. Once the phrenic nerve has been identified, the attachments of the scalenus anterior and medius muscles into the superior aspect of the first rib can be divided. These muscles can then be reflected superiorly and divided up to their origins from the transverse processes of the cervical vertebrae. This enables the majority of the muscle to be removed and detached from any surrounding tissues. Immediately, posterior to the scalenus anterior muscle lies the subclavian artery above which are the roots of the brachial plexus.

One other structure to avoid is the LTN, which arises from the body of scalenus medius muscle and proceeds laterally. Damage to this structure may cause characteristic winging of the scapula. Once the brachial plexus is clearly seen and preserved, it can be mobilized superiorly and retracted to expose the insertion of the scalenus medius muscle, which is larger in bulk than its anterior counterpart. This muscle similarly can be divided from its insertion into the first rib. The dissection again proceeds superiorly and its origins from the cervical vertebrae incised. At this point, a scalenus minimus muscle slip may be exposed, which interdigitates between the roots of the plexus. These must be divided and ideally all five roots of the plexus exposed. Scar tissue will often be identified between the roots and this must be excised posteriorly to the origin of the first rib. This procedure will enable free movement of the plexus within the canal without any extrinsic compression. Essentially, the muscle interdigitates with the plexus and causes compression of individual roots, which explains why the supraclavicular approach is optimum to achieve this and why TA surgery for first rib resection may be unsuccessful. Historically, interest in surgery for NTOS was initiated by Roos in 1966, who described the TA procedure for first rib resection.[14,17]

If a cervical rib is present then this is easily identified during the dissection. The rib is posterior to the plexus and will be seen to be displacing it anteriorly. The category of the cervical rib will decide the resection margins but a decision must be made whether to resect just the cervical rib or to combine this with a first rib resection.[7,10]

The C8 and T1 nerve roots of the brachial plexus must be protected during first rib resection to prevent trauma. Once protected, the posterior portion of the rib at the junction with the transverse process can be exposed but care must be taken to protect the thoracic nerve the more posterior the dissection. A good area to commence dissection is the inferolateral aspect of the rib. By sharply incising the intercostal muscles, a plane can be produced around the whole body of the rib and the pleura pushed downwards. The rib can be exposed anteriorly to the scalene tubercle and the bone can be excised with a rongeur forceps, commencing in a medial direction. Once soft tissue attachments have been divided, the whole of the mid portion of the rib is exposed and can be transected. Dissection of the body of the rib can proceed posteriorly to its origin ensuring complete decompression of the plexus and the subclavian artery. It is important to realize that the anterior portion of the rib can be difficult to access via the supraclavicular approach with the possibility of SV damage. One problem with the TA approach relates to exposure of vital structures. These lie deep in the operative wound and full release of the upper and lower trunks of the brachial plexus may be difficult unless in experienced hands.

VENOUS THORACIC OUTLET SYNDROME

Clinical presentation and diagnosis

Repetitive use of the arm associated with "the presence of one or more compressive elements in the thoracic outlet" may lead to thrombosis of the axillary-SV, also known as Paget–Schroetter syndrome (PSS) or effort thrombosis.[18] This typically affects males in their early 30s and is responsible for 1–4% of all cases of venous thrombosis.[12] Primary venous thrombosis of the axillo-SV presents with pain, swelling, and blue discoloration in the affected arm, and is normally diagnosed on duplex ultrasound.[19]

Cervical ribs do not usually cause compression of the SV, due to the posterior origin and anterior attachment onto the rib proximal to the vein. It is important to differentiate PSS from secondary venous thrombosis, which is related to catheters or pacemaker insertion.[12]

The extrinsic structures compressing the SV within the costoclavicular space are the subclavius muscle and a very lateral insertion of the costoclavicular ligament onto the inferior aspect of the clavicle. This can lead to extrinsic compression and ultimately wall stenosis of the SV with minimal movement **(Figure 12.3)**. As well as these there are other structures which may cause SV compression posteriorly including hypertrophied scalenus anterior muscle. The clinical outcome is extrinsic compression, which results in occlusion of the vein and thrombosis.

Management

Nonoperative management consisting of long-term anticoagulation, limb elevation, and compression stockings has significant rates of recurrence in the long term. With the modern understanding of the causes of PSS, practices have been modified and a more invasive approach has been adopted by the use of thrombolysis. The premise for this approach is the earlier clot dissolution is commenced after the initiating event the better the long-term outcomes. Following successful lysis, the cause of the venous compression can be identified and treated to optimize long-term patency rates. For acute PSS (<2 weeks after symptom onset)

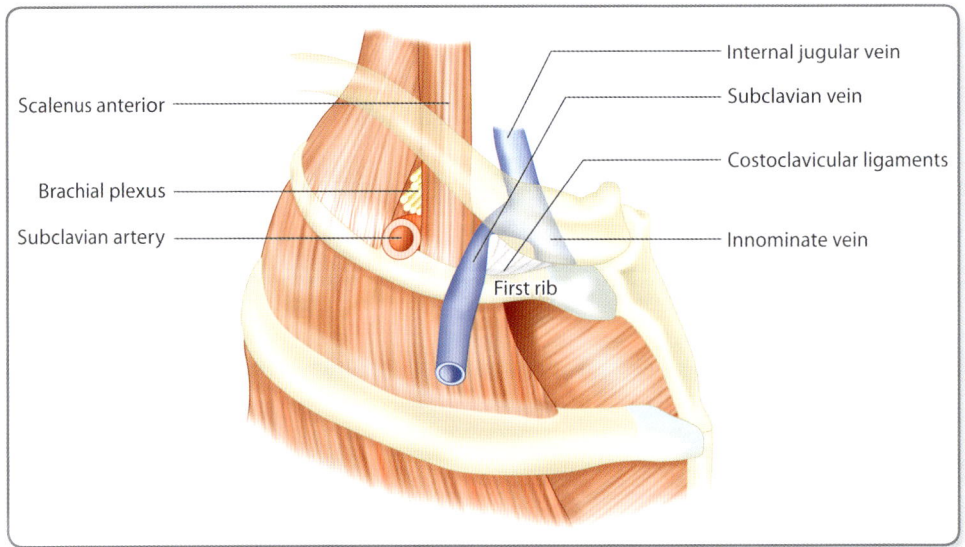

Figure 12.3 Compression of the anterior aspect of the subclavian vein as a result of abnormal lateral insertion of the costoclavicular ligament (subclavius muscle removed).

many units suggest the optimum treatment pathway is early catheter-directed thrombolysis followed by surgical decompression of the SV **(Figures 12.4A to C)**. However, after 2 weeks of thrombus being present in the SV, lysis success significantly decreases and long-term venous patency rates may be affected. Following successful thrombolysis, an intrinsic vein wall stenosis may be identified, which if left untreated may increase the risk of rethrombosis.

The place of venoplasty prior to surgical decompression is questionable, as the procedure may be a cause of further intimal damage hastening rethrombosis. Following successful thoracic outlet decompression; however, venoplasty for stenoses has been shown to aid patency rates long term.[20] The optimum timing of thoracic outlet decompression following venous lysis has never been adequately assessed by prospective trials. The early series in the literature showed a more conservative approach to decompression with some advocating an interval of up to 3 months before surgery.[21] Recent studies have shown units adopting a more aggressive approach with earlier rather than later surgery now optimum, often during the same admission following lysis.[22] Adequate decompression of the thoracic outlet should consist of complete circumferential venolysis, division of the insertion of the scalenus anterior muscle to the first rib, subclavius muscle, costoclavicular ligament, and resection of the first rib. This enables the SV to be completely mobilized circumferentially and freed from adjacent structures. Even when venolysis is undertaken within days of the thrombosis, dense scar tissue and fibrosis are often present around the vein and extending to the first rib.[23] As well as in circumferential venolysis, it is important to free the SV both proximally and distally to the stenosis.

For patients presenting with chronic PSS (>2 weeks after symptom onset), lysis is less likely to be successful and a chronic fibrotic stenotic vein wall may present. In this situation, venous reconstruction may need to be considered by using a vein patch or even an interposition graft. To ensure that this can be performed with adequate exposure, the

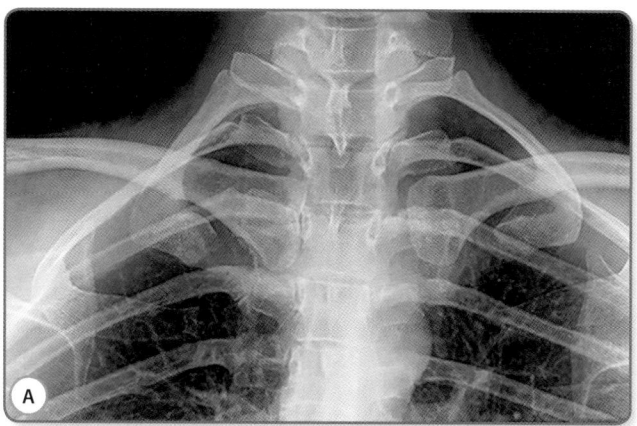

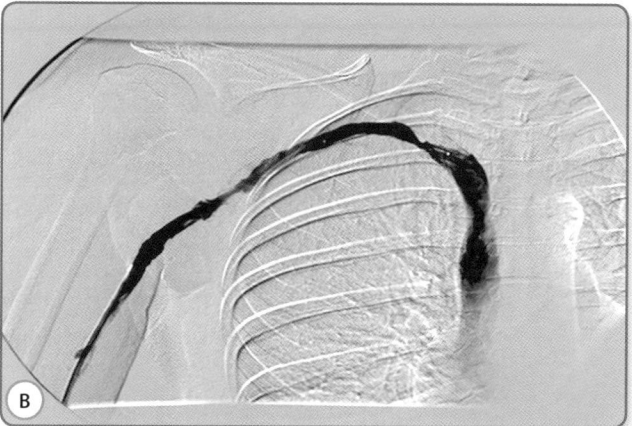

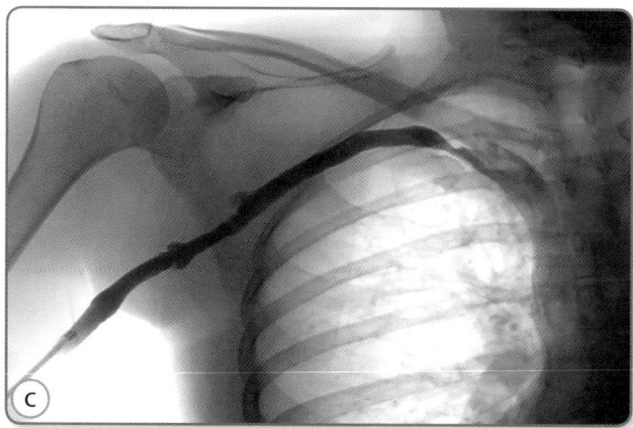

Figures 12.4A to C A 39-year-old female presenting with symptoms of right-sided Paget-Schroetter syndrome (PSS). Chest X-ray (CXR)—no evidence of cervical ribs, but abnormal "J shape" variant of first rib present bilaterally. (A) Venogram and thrombolysis of right subclavian vein (SCV) at 24 hours showing stenosis of the SCV. (B) Repeat thrombolysis at 48 hours demonstrates full lysis with persistent stenosis of the SV. (C) The patient subsequently underwent first rib resection via an infraclavicular approach.

SV needs to be dissected medially and possibly posteriorly to the manubrium. This may be technically difficult to perform by the solitary TA or supraclavicular approach without an additional IC incision.

Paget-Schroetter syndrome is relatively uncommon, which may explain the lack of RCTs comparing the various surgical approaches for thoracic decompression. Current recommendations for management of PSS are based on reviews of the literature and individual experience with the various surgical approaches. In the United Kingdom, a survey conducted of members of the Vascular Surgical Society in 2004 showed that less than two-thirds considered surgical decompression an appropriate intervention.[24] Of those in favor of surgical management, 4% performed a PC incision with 55% undergoing a TA approach, 28% opting for a supraclavicular route, and 13% preferring an axillary and supraclavicular route.[24]

Recent studies from the USA have shown that high-volume centers dealing with PSS are more likely to encompass the IC approach on its own or combined with a supraclavicular approach, in preference to the more traditional TA approach.[20,25-28] This approach has the advantage of direct access to the anterior aspect of the SV-enabling reconstruction at the time of decompression. Importantly, the risk of inadequate rib resection causing persistent external compression of the SV or damage to the venous collaterals is minimized with the IC approach.

Venous TOS patients usually benefit from 3 to 6 months of anticoagulation post-decompression. Imaging should be performed postdecompression specifically looking for vein patency and the development of stenosis in the postoperative period. Any residual SV stenosis may be suitable for venoplasty (as long as adequate decompression has been performed); however, evidence concerning the use of stents in SV stenosis has not been favorable.[25] The length of the time of anticoagulation is unknown at present but probably 3–6 months is appropriate.

ARTERIAL THORACIC OUTLET SYNDROME

Clinical presentation and diagnosis

Arterial TOS is the least common type of TOS and accounts for approximately 1% of all cases.[1] Sir Astley Cooper in 1821 was the first to describe the clinical features of arterial compression at the thoracic outlet, which may include cold peripheries, reduced or absent pulses in the affected arm, and in the chronic situation finger ulceration as a result of embolic events and ischemia.[8,29] Extrinsic compression of the subclavian artery by a cervical rib or anomalous first rib is invariably the cause for arm ischemia. Long-standing compression of the artery leads to intimal vessel damage at the compression point and poststenotic dilation. This in turn may be a cause of turbulent blood flow leading to aneurysm and thrombus formation.[8] A characteristic clinical finding is hand or digital ischemia following embolism from a mural thrombus proximally. Arterial compression may be diagnosed on duplex ultrasound, with plain X-rays being an invaluable investigation in ascertaining the presence of a cervical rib **(Figure 12.5A)**. Further investigations including angiography and CT or MR angiography can be obtained when distal embolization is apparent and arterial reconstruction a possibility after thoracic decompression **(Figures 12.5B and C)**.[6]

It is important to recognize an anomalous first rib (as opposed to a cervical rib), which may impinge on the superior aspect of the subclavian artery **(Figures 12.6A and B)**. Many with subclavian artery stenosis or aneurysms secondary to a cervical or anomalous first rib remain asymptomatic and Sanders (2002)[10] suggests that if the diameter of the dilated arterial segment is 1.5 times the diameter of the proximal artery then this is an indication for rib resection.[10]

Arterial thoracic outlet syndrome

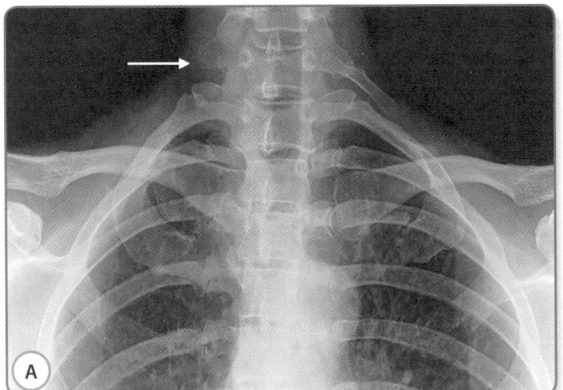
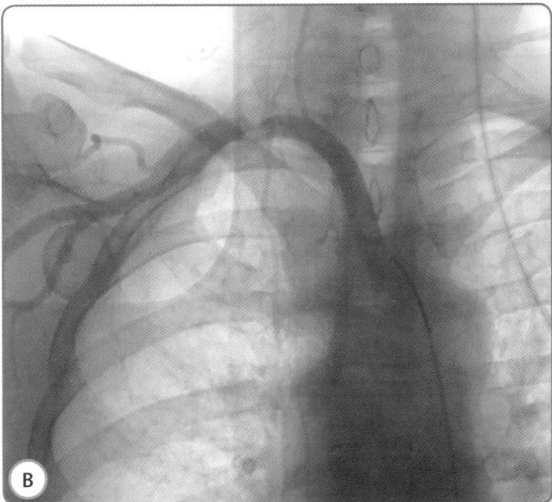
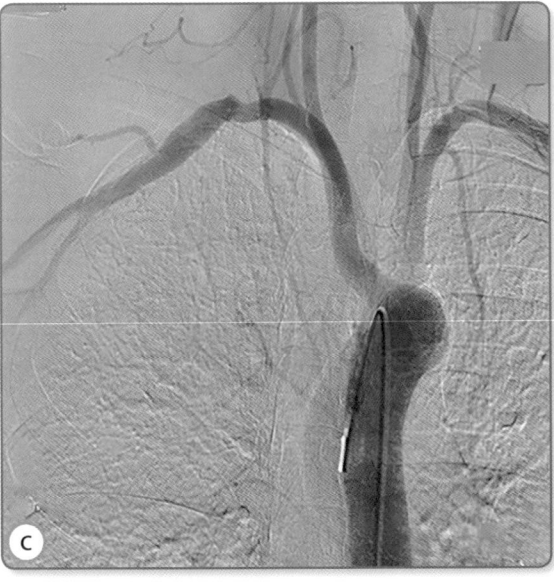

Figures 12.5A to C A 48-year-old female presenting with 3-day history of right hand ischemia, 20 years after excision of right cervical rib. (A) Chest X-ray (CXR)—left cervical rib and bony opacity above the anterior end of the right first rib (arrow) representing a residual part of a previous right cervical rib. (B) Computed tomography (CT) angiogram—indentation of right subclavian artery at the level of the first rib with mild poststenotic dilatation. (C) Poststenotic dilatation of the right subclavian artery. Incidental findings of aberrant origin of the right subclavian artery directly off the aorta and common origin of the right and left common carotid arteries.

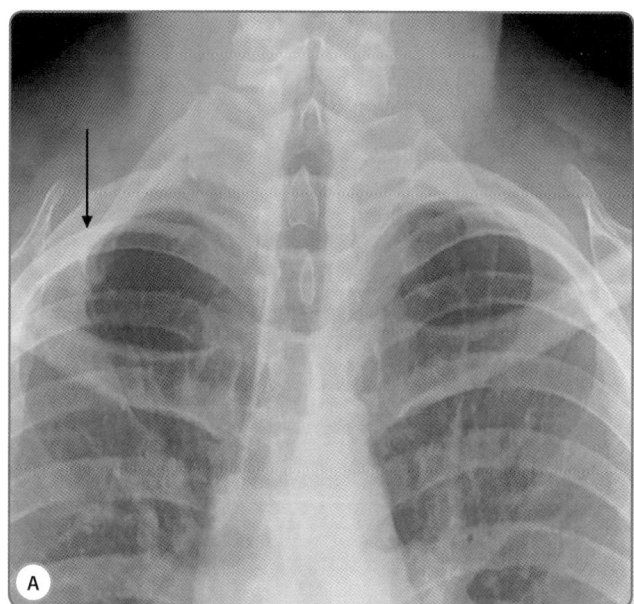
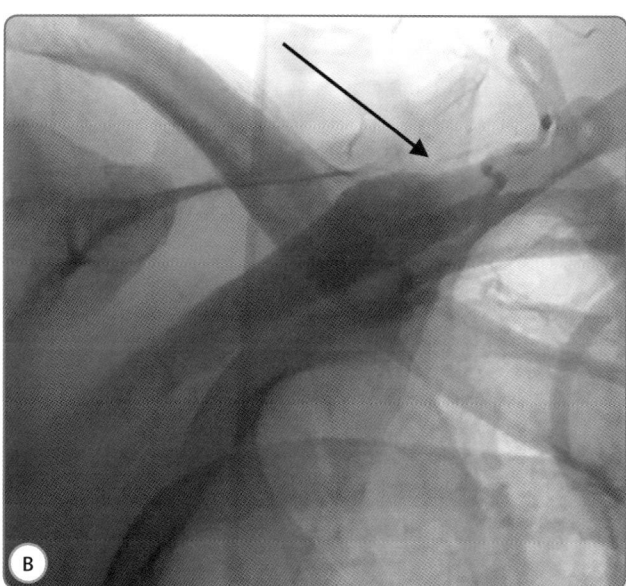

Figures 12.6A and B (A) Free floating first rib (arrow) in a 35-year-old male presenting with right upper limb ischemia. (B) Angiogram showing poststenotic dilatation distal to the point where the free end of the floating first rib pinches the superior aspect of the right subclavian artery (arrow).

Management

Surgical decompression of the axillosubclavian artery is best performed by removal of the first and cervical rib (when the latter is present), which can be done either via a TA or supraclavicular approach. However, if arterial reconstruction is necessary, the supraclavicular approach is better as access to the medial subclavian artery is excellent. Once the artery is exposed and clamps applied, an arteriotomy is performed, whereby the subclavian artery is opened and luminal debris can be removed. If the artery is thrombosed, arterial reconstruction can be performed using a vein or PTFE graft.

CONCLUSION

Over 90% of patients with TOS present with neurogenic symptoms and these patients require careful diagnosis and workup, as a significant number may undergo unnecessary surgery, if more common diagnoses such as carpal tunnel syndrome or radiculopathies have not been excluded. Early involvement of neurologists and physiotherapists is essential, in order to identify the group which may benefit from surgery after conservative measures have failed. In contrast to true NTOS, nonspecific NTOS presents with a myriad of symptoms that may not correlate with investigations or the predicted clinical picture explained by compression of the brachial plexus at the interscalene triangle and pectoralis minor space.

The early surgical approach to treat NTOS was TA and today remains a standard technique with excellent decompression achieved. The supraclavicular approach has the added advantage of allowing access to the upper roots of the brachial plexus and excision of muscle bands and scar tissue. It is difficult to assess the advantages of one of these approaches over the other in treating NTOS, as no RCTs have been performed to date.

- For venous and arterial compression, diagnosis is more straightforward, as symptoms and signs are better defined. In contrast to NTOS, early surgery is necessary for arterial and venous TOS and conservative treatment is a rare consideration nowadays. The current management of venous TOS (PSS) is catheter thrombolysis and first rib resection. The surgery usually involves the TA or PC approach. However, there is increasing literature concerning the IC approach, which enables venous reconstruction to be performed under direct vision. If a supraclavicular approach has been used then an additional IC is optimum for exposure. PSS patients usually benefit from 3 to 6 months of anticoagulation postdecompression. Any residual SV stenosis may be suitable for venoplasty, however, evidence concerning the use of stents has not been favorable.
- Arterial TOS is the least common. Arterial compression may lead to poststenotic dilatation and mural thrombus formation with the risk of distal embolization. Early diagnosis and immediate treatment are crucial to prevent complications.
- A supraclavicular approach should be used for arterial TOS, when arterial reconstruction is necessary.

> **Key points for clinical practice**
>
> - Over 90% of TOS cases are neurogenic in origin and occur in young and healthy people. Causes are cervical ribs, anomalous scalene musculature, and fascial bands which may interdigitate with the plexus roots causing extrinsic compression of the brachial plexus.
> - The distinction between "true" and "disputed" or nonspecific TOS is important, as it appears that nonspecific TOS may be overdiagnosed and more importantly, surgical treatment may not be as effective as in the case of "true" NTOS.
> - True NTOS is rare, with an estimated incidence of 1 in 1,000,000.
> - Investigations are often normal and the diagnosis of NTOS is often made by excluding other causes such as carpal tunnel syndrome and radiculopathies.
> - Initial treatment is conservative using physiotherapy, anti-inflammatory agents, and exercises to improve posture.
> - Surgery for NTOS consists of scalenectomy, cervical/first rib resection, and plexus neurolysis for bands and any anomalous scalene musculature.

- Venous thoracic outlet compression caused by PSS is a specific problem related to thrombosis of the SV secondary to compression between the first rib, clavicle, subclavius muscle, and costoclavicular ligament.
- Arterial TOS is the least common and is usually caused by a cervical or anomalous first rib causing extrinsic compression in the scalene triangle.
- While cervical ribs inserting onto the first or second rib, either directly or by a congenital band, may be easier to recognize, abnormal first ribs are an important cause of extrinsic compression at the thoracic outlet.

REFERENCES

1. Sanders RJ, Hammond SL, Rao NM. Diagnosis of thoracic outlet syndrome. J Vasc Surg. 2007;46(3):601-4.
2. Poole GV, Thomae KR. Thoracic outlet syndrome reconsidered. Am Surg. 1996;62(4):287-91.
3. Povlsen B, Hansson T, Povlsen SD. Treatment for thoracic outlet syndrome. Cochrane Database Syst Rev. 2014;11:CD007218.
4. Illig KA, Donahue D, Duncan A, et al. Reporting standards of the Society for Vascular Surgery for thoracic outlet syndrome. J Vasc Surg. 2016;64(3):e23-e35.
5. Panegyres PK, Moore N, Gibson R, et al. Thoracic outlet syndromes and magnetic resonance imaging. Brain. 1993;116(Pt 4):823-41.
6. Rigberg DA, Freischlag JA, Machleder HI. Vascular compression syndromes. In: Creager MA, Dzau V, Loscalzo J (Eds). Vascular Medicine: A Companion to Braunwald's Heart Disease, 1st edition. Philadelphia: Elsevier; 2006. pp. 920-33.
7. Chang KZ, Likes K, Davis K, et al. The significance of cervical ribs in thoracic outlet syndrome. J Vasc Surg. 2013;57(3):771-5.
8. Ferrante MA. The thoracic outlet syndromes. Muscle Nerve. 2012;45(6):780-95.
9. Nelson RM, Davis RW. Thoracic outlet compression syndrome. Ann Thorac Surg. 1969;8(5):437-51.
10. Sanders RJ, Hammond SL. Management of cervical ribs and anomalous first ribs causing neurogenic thoracic outlet syndrome. J Vasc Surg. 2002;36(1):51-6.
11. Coote H. Exostosis of the left transverse process of the seventh cervical vertebra, surrounded by blood vessels and nerves: successful removal. Lancet. 1861;1;360-1.
12. Illig KA, Doyle AJ. A comprehensive review of Paget-Schroetter syndrome. J Vasc Surg. 2010;51(6):1538-47.
13. Roos DB. The thoracic outlet syndrome is underrated. Arch Neurol. 1990;47:327-8.
14. Wilbourn AJ. Thoracic outlet syndrome surgery causing severe brachial plexopathy. Muscle Nerve. 1988;11(1):66-74.
15. Le Forestier N, Mouton P, Maisonobe T, et al. True neurological thoracic outlet syndrome: 10 cases. J Peripher Nerv Syst. 2000;5(4):238.
16. Jordan SE, Machleder HI. Diagnosis of thoracic outlet syndrome using electrophysiologically guided anterior scalene blocks. Ann Vasc Surg. 1998;12(3):260-4.
17. Wood VE, Ellison DW. Results of upper plexus thoracic outlet syndrome operation. Ann Thorac Surg. 1994;58(2):458-61.
18. Urschel HC Jr, Kourlis H Jr. Thoracic outlet syndrome: a 50-year experience at Baylor University Medical Center. Proc (Bayl Univ Med Cent). 2007;20(2):125-35.
19. Molina JE, Hunter DW, Dietz CA. Protocols for Paget-Schroetter syndrome and late treatment of chronic subclavian vein obstruction. Ann Thorac Surg. 2009;87(2):416-22.
20. Maxey TS, Reece B, Ellman PI, et al. Safety and efficacy of the supraclavicular approach to thoracic outlet decompression. Ann Thorac Surg. 2003;76(2):396-400.
21. Machleder HI. Evaluation of a new treatment strategy for Paget-Schroetter syndrome: spontaneous thrombosis of the axillary-subclavian vein. J Vasc Surg. 1993;17(2):305-15.
22. Angle N, Gelebert HA, Farooq MM, et al. Safety and efficacy of early surgical decompression of the thoracic outlet for Paget-Schroetter syndrome. Ann Vasc Surg. 2001;15(1):37-42.
23. Thompson RW, Schneider PA, Nelken NA, et al. Circumferential venolysis and paraclavicular thoracic outlet decompression for "effort thrombosis" of the subclavian vein. J Vasc Surg. 1992;16(5):723-32.
24. Khan SN, Stansby G. Current management of Paget-Schroetter syndrome in the UK. Ann R Coll Surg Engl. 2004;86(1):29-34.

25. Azakie A, McElhinney DB, Thompson RW, et al. Surgical management of subclavian-vein effort thrombosis as a result of thoracic outlet compression. J Vasc Surg. 1998;28(5):777-86.
26. Vasu Divi BA, Proctor MC, Axelrod DA, et al. Thoracic outlet decompression for subclavian vein thrombosis. Arch Surg. 2005;140(1):54-7.
27. Stone DH, Scali ST, Bjerk AA, et al. Aggressive treatment of idiopathic axillo-subclavian vein thrombosis provides excellent long-term function. J Vasc Surg. 2010;52(1):127-31.
28. Schneider DB, Dimuzio PJ, Martin ND, et al. Combination treatment of venous thoracic outlet syndrome: Open surgical decompression and intraoperative angioplasty. J Vasc Surg. 2004;40(4):599-603.
29. Roos DB. Historical perspectives and anatomic considerations. Thoracic outlet syndrome. Semin Thorac Cardiovasc Surg. 1996;8(2):183-9.

Section 9

Innovation in Surgery

CHAPTER

13. The Use of Three-dimensional Printing in Surgery

Chapter 13

The use of three-dimensional printing in surgery

Joseph Hardwicke

INTRODUCTION

Traditional manufacturing may be considered a "subtractive" technique, with the final form being tooled or molded from a larger piece of material. This can be done by many techniques including milling, injection molding, carving or using a computer numerical control router. Three-dimensional (3D) printing is an "additive" technique in which successive layers of material can be created and stacked to create a final form, with the individual layers digitally designed from a 3D image source file. It is also referred to as rapid prototyping or additive manufacturing. 3D printing gives engineers the ability to prototype and manufacture customized end-use products, as well as reducing assembly costs, and can serve as a cost-effective low volume production process. Such technology has rapidly penetrated the medical device industry, with applications such as patient-specific implants for reconstruction of the skull and facial skeleton, hip and knee prostheses, and scaffolds for tissue engineering being developed.[1-3] It may play a significant role in the future of surgical custom-made implants, therapeutics and prostheses.

Additive manufacturing processes were established during the 1980s with the advent of photo-hardening polymers that could be activated by UV light to create forms, but did not initially rely on the layer-by-layer deposition process.[4] Alain Le Méhauté, Olivier de Witte and Jean Claude André in France, and Chuck Hull in the USA, independently developed the additive layer process, or stereolithography, in 1984, with Hill being awarded a US Patent in 1986.[5] It was Hill who defined the process as a "system for generating 3D objects by creating a cross-sectional pattern of the object to be formed" and pioneered the STereoLithography (STL; .stl) file format, which is in common usage today.[6,7]

As image capture, computational power and printing accuracy has increased, the ability to produce complex and intricate 3D structures has now surpassed that of traditional subtractive manufacturing. With a reduction on the costs of hardware, software and consumables, 3D printing is available to all, from the hobbyist, to the multinational medical devices industry. In this review, the manufacturing processes will be explained, as well as the many medical applications to which it may become commonplace.

THREE-DIMENSIONAL PRINTING METHODOLOGY

The essence of 3D printing for surgical applications is the acquisition of patient-specific digital image data followed by post-acquisition manipulation of the digital form, which can then be printed.

Image capture and processing

In the printing of 3D forms for surgical applications, the most common methodology for image capture is using existing medical imaging platforms, such as high-resolution CT, ultrasound or MRI, that can capture the structure of intracorporeal structures. The Digital Imaging and Communications in Medicine (DICOM) format is a standard for handling, storing, printing, and transmitting information in medical imaging and consists of a number of attributes, including patient identification information which is inextricably linked to the image file. From such file information, a sequential series of tomogram slices can be transformed into a discrete volumetric 3D representation, within appropriate viewer software.

For external surfaces and extracorporeal structures, 3D scanners may be used to capture the image detail in a contact or non-contact methodology. Contact scanners require contact with the object being scanned, and as such the act of scanning the object might modify, desterilize or damage it. Contact scanning is not common place for medical or surgical applications of 3D scanning. Non-contact active scanners emit a form of radiation or light and detect its reflection or radiation passing through an object in order to probe an object or environment. The most commonly employed technology is the time-of-flight laser scanner. At the heart of this type of scanner is a laser range finder, designed to calculate the distance of a surface by timing the round-trip time of a pulse of light. The laser range finder only detects the distance of one point in its direction of view and so the scanner collects data in its entire field of view one point at a time by changing the range finder's direction of view to scan different points. The subject of the scan may also be rotated in three dimensions to allow capture of the entire surface structure. Typical time-of-flight 3D laser scanners can measure the distance of 10,000–100,000 points every second.

After acquisition of this 3D data source file, open source software can be then used to produce a 3D mesh, which can then be manipulated, converted and exported in a format compatible with proprietary 3D printers. The industry standard file format is .stl which describes a triangulated surface using a 3D Cartesian coordinate system (x, y, z). Computer-aided design (CAD) software can then be employed to manipulate, resize and render a component of the original file, for example to create a custom-made prosthesis. The number of triangles used in its construction and the computer processing power available will only limit the detail and size of the file. When an appropriate digital form has been created it can be exported to a compatible 3D printing platform.

- Conventional medical imaging software and hardware can be used to produce a digital 3D representation of an intracorporeal structure.
- Time-of-flight laser scanning may be employed in the image capture of external surface features.
- The raw image file can be manipulated post acquisition by CAD and exported to a suitable 3D printing platform for rapid prototyping.

Printing

Various methods for the sequential deposition of materials have been developed. At the core of the concept is the ability to manipulate the printable substrate, from a semi-liquid or powder state, to a solid or semi-solid that can then be stacked in a controllable manner.

Extrusion

The most familiar 3D printing technique to the hobbyist or small-scale 3D printing concern is extrusion. Fused deposition modeling (FDM) uses a heated semi-solid thermoplastic that is forced through an extrusion nozzle at a controlled rate, whilst being moved on a 3D armature. The printing substrate then cools to become a solid to allow sequential stacking. More recently a hand-held "pen" has been developed to allow a free form of variant of 3D printing.[8] Typical thermoplastics that are used are acrylonitrile butadiene styrene (ABS), polylactic acid, polyamide and polycarbonate. This technique is suitable for producing teaching models and implants, but not for printing of cell-based scaffolds due to the high temperatures (over 100°C) involved. Direct-write bioprinting utilizes the same mechanics of extrusion and movement of the printer head, but a more viscous gel substrate can be used that does not require an additional action (e.g., cooling) at the time of printing to allow stacking of layers, although secondary cross-linking may be required to produce a more solid final form.[9]

Light polymerization

Stereolithography (STL) was the first 3D printing methodology to be patented and is based upon laser light that is focused onto a vat of liquid photopolymer resin. The photopolymer resins consist of a mixture monomer and oligomer subunits and photoinitiator molecules, and when exposed to UV light (or visible light) undergo chain-growth polymerization and cross-linking. Polyjet 3D printing uses a photopolymer but rather than using a vat, the process uses similar technology to ink jet printing, with multiple colours of photopolymer instantly cured after printing.[10] The properties of the photocured material can be tailored according to the type of monomer (styrene, acrylate, N-vinylpyrolidone) and the addition of functionalized oligomers (epoxides, urethanes, polyesters) to provide flexibility, adhesion or chemical resistance. The speed of cure and density of cross-linking can also be manipulated though the composition of the resin. Again, after an initial layer is photocured and subsequent layers are printed on top to produce a final 3D form. Due to the cytoxicity of the substrates, this technique is not usually suitable for cell-based constructs.

Powder bed

Selective laser sintering (SLS) is similar to STL, but is based upon a powder rather than a liquid. A pulsed laser selectively fuses small particles of plastic, metal, ceramic or glass to produce an additive 3D form. In contrast to other additive manufacturing processes, it does not require additional physical supports to aid printing of overhanging designs (e.g. if trying to print an inverted cone), as the unsintered material provides this. Selective laser melting is a comparable technique but takes the substrate material to its melting point, rather than the lower temperature required for sintering.

- Forced deposition modeling is an extrusion printing technique, based upon an armature that can be controlled in three dimensions. As the printed liquid polymer cools and solidifies successive layers of print to be combined into a fully 3D form.
- Stereolithography requires a variably focused laser to initiate a polymeric chain reaction to produce a solid 3D structure from a liquid resin, whilst SLS uses laser energy to fuse a powder substrate in a similar manner. Polyjet printing uses ink jet technology that is instantly cured after printing.
- For printing of biological 3D forms, consideration must be made about the temperature and toxicity of the printing process.

Bioinks and bioprinting

The majority of applications of 3D printing in surgery in the present day are in the production of custom made forms for teaching, implantation or prostheses. These do not require biological components such as cells, matrix proteins or cytokines. A printing substrate that has biological components can be referred to as a bioink[11] and although the previously mentioned image acquisition and processing methods can be used for designing 3D constructs, specific consideration has to be made to the bioprinting process. Biological components may not tolerate the high temperatures and pressures of traditional 3D printing, and the matrix that will form the 3D structure, as well as any polymerization or cross-linking agents, will need to avoid or limit cytotoxicity. Such printing methods must also be performed in a humidity-controlled sterile environment with consideration for disease communication. To mimic complex extracellular matrix structures in vitro, cell-laden hydrogels have been printed with plans for future clinical translation.

Numerous ethical challenges are raised by efforts to repopulate 3D scaffolds designed to remain inside the body with functioning cells. Mandatory transparency about the techniques involved, cell sources, financial and physical costs to patients, strategies for dealing with experimental failure, and the ability to assist patients after initial treatment are necessary.[12]

Bioinks

Many different cell types have been used as a component of a bioink, including fibroblasts,[13] mesenchymal stem cells,[14] hepatocytes[15] and neuronal cells.[16] To allow cellular metabolism within the scaffold, hydrogels are most commonly used alone, or in combination. Hydrogels consist of a network of natural or synthetic polymer chains that are hydrophilic, in which water is the dispersion medium. They act as a mimic of the extracellular matrix. Hydrogels that can be used as a bioink substrate include natural polymers such as alginate, agarose, gelatin, collagen, fibrin, hyaluronic acid, silk and chitosan;[17] and synthetic polymers including polyethylene glycol and block co-polymers such as Pluronic gels.[18] All can be functionalized and customized to allow adjustment of the viscosity to allow extrusion and printing with the production of a solid, or semi-solid form. The viability of the component cells is proportional to the distance of the cells from the nutrient supply. To improve cellular survival, vascular-like networks have been printed within larger volumetric constructs,[19] although the higher resolution printing techniques such as STL may be required. For the application of 3D bioprinting to surgery, such as synthetic organ fabrication, larger constructs will be required with an intrinsic, custom-fabricated vascular network.

Direct-write bioprinting

Direct-write systems are a variant of extrusion printing and are designed to dispense the materials in layered lines onto a stage using a single syringe or multiple syringes.[9] Unlike FDM and other extrusion techniques, the higher non-biological temperatures can be avoided, or at least limited in intensity and duration. A higher viscosity substrate is used that can be extruded but will retain its structural integrity at biological temperatures to allow stacking of layers, without the need for an immediate curing process. Three methods of direct writing can be used: pneumatic, mechanical, and a pneumatic-mechanical hybrid.[9,20,21] The pressures required to extrude the viscous gel are applied through either a high-pressure gas source, or a mechanical worm screw to activate the syringe driver system. The pneumatic systems work better with high viscosity materials, while mechanical systems are better suited in working with materials of low viscosity.

In order to create gels of higher viscosity, capable of extrusion and stacking without an intrinsic thickening process at time of printing can be done by the addition of thickening agents[22] which can then later be leeched form the final form, higher concentration of the gelling agent in solution or partial cross-linking of polymer gel, prior to a final completion cross-linking step when the final printed form is complete.
- Bioprinting takes advantage of suspended or encapsulated cells within a water-laden scaffold to produce in vitro models of tissues, or 3D forms capable of clinical translation.
- Bioinks contain biological components within a gel matrix that is viscous enough to extrude and stack layers to create a 3D form.
- Direct-write bioprinting employs an extrusion-based system, either mechanical or pneumatic, to create a 3D structure. The bioink undergoes a secondary step to produce a stabilized final form.
- Cellular metabolism is limited by diffusion of nutrients through the gel matrix and as such, at present, there is a size limitation of the structures that can be produced.

APPLICATIONS

Surgical teaching and training

One of the areas of medicine and surgery that has readily taken up 3D printing is teaching and training. Rather than traditional anatomical models that have been used over the last two centuries, individual models based upon unique pathology can be designed and printed from patient imaging studies. Rapid prototyping is an evolving technology that has the potential to revolutionize medical education.

Three-dimensional printing has been used to create personalized, patient-specific, hepatic models for surgical trainee education. Patient-specific 3D models of portal and hepatic venous anatomy have been printed using SLS at a cost of less than US $100 per model.[23] Other structures such as complex intracranial aneurysms, cleft lip and palates, free flaps and the renal vasculature have also been printed in a using STL or polyjet.[24-27] Although soft tissues can be mimicked using FDM, STL and SLS, hard tissues such as the bicortical calvarial bone can be produced from plaster composite using a powder bed technique.[28] These models can allow the trainees' visual and tactile senses to work in unison, providing a more extensive understanding, which can be translated to the operating theatre. Ultimately, low-cost disposable models could allow surgeons-in-training to dissect the models and discard them once the techniques have been mastered.

Patient information

As well as surgical training, 3D modeling has the capacity to create models of a patient's individual anatomic deformity and serve as an indispensable tool when educating patients. If patients can hold a printed model and compare it with a model of their postoperative outcome, they may more realistically manage their expectations.[29] An individual 3D Polyjet-printed model of a kidney tumor has been shown to improve understanding of basic kidney physiology, kidney anatomy, tumor characteristics and the planned surgical procedure.[30]

Operative planning

For surgical planning, 3D-printed patient-specific models have been used to enhance understanding complex procedures and improve the efficiency and cost-effectiveness of the operating procedure. Preoperative review of the 3D model can allow the surgeon to anticipate intraoperative difficulties, selection of optimal surgical approach and the need for specific equipment.[31] In preoperative planning, 3D-printing has been used to aid craniofacial reconstruction;[32] skull base and cervical spine reconstruction;[33] mapping of congenital heart defects and tracheobronchial anomalies in cardiothoracic surgery and cardiac transplantation;[34,35] modeling of aortic dissection in vascular surgery;[36] partial nephrectomy for renal tumors in urology;[37] reconstruction of frontal sinus defects in ear, nose, and throat surgery;[38] treatment of wounds in plastic surgery;[39] and liver transplantation in general surgery.[40] Furthermore, patient-specific surgical templates and jigs to have been used in maxillofacial surgery, neurosurgery, orthopedic surgery, hand surgery, and general surgery to enhance the intraoperative process.[31]

Implants

Synthetic implants

One of the first clinical applications of 3D printed medical implants has been in the field of craniomaxillofacial reconstruction and orthopedics. Vertebral, hip, pelvis, and mandibular implants have been produced with the use of 3D-printed plastic and titanium implants.[41] Tissue-engineered bone grafts are based upon synthetic and scaffolds have been used for bone regeneration, thus negating the need for a donor source and the associated donor-site morbidity. Synthetically produced scaffolds may not precisely mimic the biochemical or structural properties of the native scaffold but allow for greater control in their fabrication process and more reliable reproducibility. The material properties, bioactivity, porosity, and shape of synthetic grafts can be closely controlled and customized for specific applications.

Bioprinting

Biologic scaffolds may provide an alternative to autologous tissue grafting or microvascular tissue flap transfer. Bone tissue engineering may provide alternatives to inorganic implants by using biocompatible scaffold materials and autologous cells. Once the scaffold is shaped to form an identical model of the original bone or joint, it can then seeded with mesenchymal stem cells isolated from the patient's bone marrow or fat tissue.[42] The new bone is either incubated in vivo in the patient or placed into a bioreactor for maturation. As well as avoiding the need for a suitable bone graft donor site with the resulting comorbidities, and the size restrictions of traditional bone graft harvesting, autologous reconstruction using a 3D printed scaffold may have improved longevity and reduced complications.

Soft-tissue structures have also been developed in vitro including cell-laden scaffolds to replace heart valves,[22] cartilage scaffolds for ear and nose reconstruction, and skin composites.[43] A scaffold-based approach relies on temporary scaffolds to facilitate cellular attachment, metabolism and proliferation, followed by cellular secretion of extracellular matrix to remodel the surrounding environment. With degradation of the printed scaffold over time, and replacement by autologous tissues, complications that can be associated with permanent scaffolds such as implant extrusion or infection may be avoided.

Prostheses

The ability to create individually-customized prosthetic devices has led to the rapid development of additive manufacturing in this area of rehabilitation medicine. Prostheses including artificial ears, noses, eyes and limbs can be modeled on unaffected anatomy, such as a normal contralateral structure, and printed. Multiple open-source 3D hand designs are currently available online to allow users to print a dynamic hand prosthesis, using existing FDM technology. The majority of available designs share common elements such as an anthropomorphic appearance, with articulated joints linked to a forearm gauntlet. The tenodesis effect is employed to create composite grasp powered by wrist motion and passive digital release via elastic components. The aim of these projects is to increase the availability of complex prosthesis to the world and decrease the procurement costs. This is most valid in the pediatric age group as multiple prostheses will be required to keep up with normal growth, and as such, costs can be prohibitive.[44]

- Patient-specific models can be created from DICOM data using 3-D printing to allow spatial appreciation of complex structures for teaching and patient education.
- Operative planning, including the production of surgical jigs, customized drill-guides and instrumentation may improve efficiency.
- Custom-made implants can be rapidly produced and may, in the future, replace the need for autologous donor tissues.
- Low-cost prosthesis can be produced to improve patient rehabilitation, form and function after surgery.

REGULATIONS

To reach the general market, a medical device must first pass a set of standards set by the appropriate body. In the US, the Food and Drug Administration (FDA) classifies devices based on risk of the new device and the level of control necessary to assure safety and efficacy. Class I devices are considered low-risk while Class III devices, which includes most implants, are considered high-risk and require premarket approval. They are typically granted an initial investigational device exemption allowing use of the device exclusively in a FDA-regulated clinical trial to collect necessary premarket safety and efficacy information. As of December 2015, over 85 3D printed products had gained approval, including instrumentation, synthetic implants and external prostheses.[45]

Despite appropriate quality controls for printing processes, variations in manufactured devices may still occur. Each of the multistep processes of 3D printing from image capture and processing, material selection, printing, and post-printing finishing, validating and testing, may require a form of approval. The material utilized and the size and shape of the device often determines the specific techniques chosen for quality assurance testing. After printing, cleaning 3D-printed devices is necessary regardless of the 3D printing technique used: the method of cleaning varies based on the printing process employed, from removal of support materials to removal of residual monomers and other chemicals. Validation is also required to show that this finishing process does not alter the overall structure or mechanical properties of the device.

For implants, the International Organization of Standards (ISO) has published a set of standards for evaluating the biocompatibility of materials used in the manufacture of medical devices, collectively termed ISO 10993.[46] Unique factors arise when attempting to apply these standards to 3D-printed implants: materials may be altered by the various printing processes and any additives used during the manufacturing process (e.g. cross-linking agents) may also need to be tested to ensure they are removed completely during cleaning processes or that they are ISO 10993 compliant if still present within the final device. For biodegradable implants such as bioprinted forms, it is important to fully characterize the degradation profile in vitro and in vivo. Degradation studies may also be necessary for shelf life testing of final manufactured devices.[47]

Sterility is fundamental to minimizing risk of infection associated with implantable medical devices. Given the numerous materials utilized in 3D printing (both biological and non-biological), multiple-step sterilization processes may be required, depending upon compatibility between the process and device material. Sterility assurance level (SAL) is the probability of a single unit being non-sterile after it has been subjected to sterilization. In general, devices manufactured by 3D printing are subject to the same regulatory requirements for SAL and post-manufacture processing as non-3D printed devices.

- The FDA has approved 3D devices for use in humans.
- The multiple step process of 3D printing and multiple raw materials involved may require regulation at each stage.
- Devices manufactured by 3D printing are subject to the same regulatory requirements as non-3D printed devices.

SUMMARY

The role of 3D printing in surgery is expanding, and in the future may only be limited by the imagination of engineers, biomedical scientists and surgeons. At present, the main limitations are the size of the printing platform and thus the size of the 3D form that can be produced. For surgical uses, large-scale models and devices are probably not required and so this should not hold back the development. With the acceptance of the technology by regulatory agencies, and approvals being given, 3D printed products are already to market. Although the technology is expanding at great speed, regulation is still required to govern the manufacturing process to ensure that the multistage process and mixture of raw ingredients does not increase the risk of adverse events after clinical translation.

For bioprinting to succeed and provide a viable alternative to autogenous donor tissue, scaffolds need to be manufactured to include an effective vascular-like network to provide cellular nutrition. At present, the process of diffusion though a water-laden hydrogel matrix limits the size and efficacy of the printed product. To date, the most successful application of 3D printing is in the areas of surgical planning and education. With the ability to rapidly produce a unique model of an internal pathology, time and money can be saved in the operating theatre by pre-fabricating custom-implants, aiding instrument selection and optimizing the surgical approach. Possibly the next area for expansion is in the world of prosthetics and rehabilitation, with individual prostheses printed "at will" to account for the natural attrition of the prosthetic, growth of the user and upgrading the device. The emerging technology of 3D printing has the opportunity to revolutionize surgery, and make what once where cost-limited technologies available to all.

> **Key points for clinical practice**
> - Conventional medical imaging can be used to transfer unique patient data to 3D modeling software, with which a custom-made 3D model can be designed.
> - Various 3D printing methodologies are available, and can be selected based upon the design for the object that is to be printed and the materials involved.
> - Substrates for 3D printing can be specifically tailored to fulfill to optimum design requirements, such as strength, flexibility and biocompatibility.

- Light-activated photopolymers, ceramics, metals, thermoplastics, glass and natural polymers such as alginate, gelatin, collagen, fibrin, hyaluronic acid, silk and chitosan have all been used for 3D printing.
- Bioinks contain living cells and are usually based upon water-laden hydrogel structures and could potentially replace autologous tissues in the future.
- The majority of 3D printing applications that are currently used in surgery are for training, patient education and preoperative planning.
- Low-cost prosthesis can be produced to improve patient rehabilitation, form and function after surgery. Designs can be downloaded for free.
- Implantable devices require strict regulation through all stages of development, from design to manufacture to post-production quality assurance and testing.
- Devices manufactured by 3D printing are subject to the same regulatory requirements as non-3D printed devices. The FDA has approved over 85 printed devices.
- The emerging technology of 3D printing has the opportunity to revolutionize surgery, and make what once where cost-limited technologies available to all.

REFERENCES

1. Gross BC, Erkal JL, Lockwood SY, et al. Evaluation of 3D printing and its potential impact on biotechnology and the chemical sciences. Anal Chem. 2014;86(7):3240-53.
2. Klein GT, Lu Y, Wang MY. 3D printing and neurosurgery—ready for prime time? World Neurosurg. 2013;80(3-4):233-5.
3. Banks J. Adding value in additive manufacturing: researchers in the United Kingdom and Europe look to 3D printing for customization. IEEE Pulse. 2013;4(6):22-6.
4. SPIE-Professional. (2013)# Chuck Hull: Pioneer in Stereolithography. [online] Available from http://spie.org/x91418.xml. [Accessed September, 2017].
5. Hull CW. Apparatus for production of three-dimensional objects by stereolithography. Alexandria: US Patent Office; 1989.
6. 3D Systems. (2016)# 30 Years of Innovation. [online] Available from http://www.3dsystems.com/30-years-innovation. [Accessed September, 2017].
7. Chua CK, Leong KF, Lim CS. Rapid Prototyping: Principles and Applications, 3rd edition. Singapore: World Scientific Publishing Co.; 2010.
8. The3doodler. What will you create? [online] Available from http://the3doodler.com. [Accessed September, 2017].
9. Smith CM, Stone AL, Parkhill RL, et al. Three-dimensional bioassembly tool for generating viable tissue-engineered constructs. Tissue Eng. 2004;10(9-10):1566-76.
10. Ionita CN, Mokin M, Varble N, et al. Challenges and limitations of patient-specific vascular phantom fabrication using 3D Polyjet printing. Proc SPIE Int Soc Opt Eng. 2014;9038:90380M.
11. Jia J, Richards DJ, Pollard S. Engineering alginate as bioink for bioprinting. Acta Biomater. 2014;10(10):4323-31.
12. Badylak SF, Weiss DJ, Caplan A, et al. Engineered whole organs and complex tissues. Lancet. 2012;379(9819):943-52.
13. Lee V, Singh G, Trasatti JP, et al. Design and fabrication of human skin by three-dimensional bioprinting. Tissue Eng Part C Methods. 2014;20(6):473-84.
14. Liu A, Xue GH, Sun M, et al. 3D printing surgical implants at the clinic: a experimental study on anterior cruciate ligament reconstruction. Sci Rep. 2016;6:21704.
15. Bertassoni LE, Cardoso JC, Manoharan V, et al. Direct-write bioprinting of cell-laden methacrylated gelatin hydrogels. Biofabrication. 2014;6(2):024105.
16. Gu Q, Tomaskovic-Crook E, Lozano R. Functional 3D neural mini-tissues from printed gel-based bioink and human neural stem cells. Adv Healthc Mater. 2016;5(12):1429-38.

17. Gasperini L, Mano JF, Reis RL. Natural polymers for the microencapsulation of cells. J R Soc Interface. 2014;11(100):20140817.
18. Müller M, Becher J, Schnabelrauch M, et al. Nanostructured pluronic hydrogels as bioinks for 3D bioprinting. Biofabrication. 2015;7(3):035006.
19. Takei T, Sakai S, Yoshida M. In vitro formation of vascular-like networks using hydrogels. J Biosci Bioeng. #2016;122(5):519-27.
20. Smith CM1, Christian JJ, Warren WL, et al. Characterizing environmental factors that impact the viability of tissue-engineered constructs fabricated by a direct-write bioassembly tool. Tissue Eng. 2007;13(2):373-83.
21. Mironov V, Visconti RP, Kasyanov V, et al. Organ printing: tissue spheroids as building blocks. Biomaterials. 2009;30(12):2164-74.
22. Duan B, Hockaday LA, Kang KH, et al. 3D bioprinting of heterogeneous aortic valve conduits with alginate/gelatin hydrogels. J Biomed Mater Res A. 2013;101(5):1255-64.
23. Watson RA. A low-cost surgical application of additive fabrication. J Surg Educ. 2014;71(1):14-7.
24. Vakharia VN, Vakharia NN, Hill CS. Review of 3-dimensional printing on cranial neurosurgery simulation training. World Neurosurg. 2016;88:188-98.
25. Calonge WM, AlAli AB, Griffin M, et al. Three-dimensional printing of models of cleft lip and palate. Plast Reconstr Surg Glob Open. 2016;4(4):e689.
26. Mehta S, Byrne N, Karunanithy N, et al. 3D printing provides unrivalled bespoke teaching tools for autologous free flap breast reconstruction. J Plast Reconstr Aesthet Surg. 2016;69(4):578-80.
27. Kusaka M, Sugimoto M, Fukami N, et al. Initial experience with a tailor-made simulation and navigation program using a 3-D printer model of kidney transplantation surgery. Transplant Proc. 2015;47(3):596-9.
28. Tai BL, Rooney D, Stephenson F, et al. Development of a 3D-printed external ventricular drain placement simulator: technical note. J Neurosurg. 2015;123(4):1070-6.
29. Gerstle TL, Ibrahim AM, Kim PS, et al. A plastic surgery application in evolution: three-dimensional printing. Plast Reconstr Surg. 2014;133(2):446-51.
30. Bernhard JC, Isotani S, Matsugasumi T, et al. Personalized 3D printed model of kidney and tumor anatomy: a useful tool for patient education. World J Urol. 2016;34(3):337-45.
31. Eltorai AE, Nguyen E, Daniels AH. Three-dimensional printing in orthopedic surgery. Orthopedics. 2015;38(11):684-7.
32. Steinbacher DM. Three-dimensional analysis and surgical planning in craniomaxillofacial surgery. J Oral Maxillofac Surg. 2015;73(12):S40-56.
33. Pacione D, Tanweer O, Berman P, et al. The utility of a multimaterial 3D printed model for surgical planning of complex deformity of the skull base and craniovertebral junction. J Neurosurg. 2016;125(5):1194-7.
34. Kurup HK, Samuel BP, Vettukattil JJ. Hybrid 3D printing: a game-changer in personalized cardiac medicine? Expert Rev Cardiovasc Ther. 2015;13(12):1281-4.
35. Giannopoulos AA, Steigner ML, George E, et al. Cardiothoracic applications of 3-dimensional printing. J Thorac Imaging. 2016;31(5):253-72.
36. Hossien A, Gesomino S, Maessen J, et al. The interactive use of multi-dimensional modeling and 3D printing in preplanning of type a aortic dissection. J Card Surg. 2016;31(7):441-5.
37. Zhang Y, Ge HW, Li NC, et al. Evaluation of three-dimensional printing for laparoscopic partial nephrectomy of renal tumors: a preliminary report. World J Urol. 2016;34(4):533-7.
38. Daniel M, Watson J, Hoskison E, et al. Frontal sinus models and onlay templates in osteoplastic flap surgery. J Laryngol Otol. 2011;125(1):82-5.
39. Kamali P, Dean D, Skoracki R, et al. The current role of three-dimensional printing in plastic surgery. Plast Reconstr Surg. 2016;137(3):1045-55.
40. Zein NN, Hanouneh IA, Bishop PD, et al. Three-dimensional print of a liver for preoperative planning in living donor liver transplantation. Liver Transpl. 2013;19(12):1304-10.
41. Bauermeister AJ, Zuriarrain A, Newman MI. Three-dimensional printing in plastic and reconstructive surgery: A systematic review. Ann Plast Surg. 2016;77(5):569-76.
42. Temple JP, Hutton DL, Hung BP, et al. Engineering anatomically shaped vascularized bone grafts with hASCs and 3D-printed PCL scaffolds. J Biomed Mater Res A. 2014;102(12):4317-25.
43. Ng WL, Wang S, Yeong WY, et al. Skin bioprinting: impending reality or fantasy? Trends Biotechnol. 2016;34(9):689-99.
44. Burn MB, Ta A, Gogola GR. Three-dimensional printing of prosthetic hands for children. J Hand Surg Am. 2016;41(5):e103-9.

45. US Food and Drug Administration. (2013). 3D Printing of Medical Devices. [online] Available from http://www.fda.gov/MedicalDevices/ProductsandMedicalProcedures/3DPrintingofMedicalDevices/default.htm. [Accessed September, 2017].
46. International Organization for Standardization. 2013 Biological evaluation of medical devices (ISO/IEC JTC 1. ISO/IEC 10993). Geneva/Switzerl: ISO/IEC; 2013.
47. Morrison RJ, Kashlan KN, Flanangan CL, et al. Regulatory considerations in the design and manufacturing of implantable 3D-printed medical devices. Clin Transl Sci. 2015;8(5):594-600.

Section 10

Clinical Trials

CHAPTER

14. A Review of Recent Randomized Controlled Trials in Surgery

Chapter 14

A review of recent randomized controlled trials in surgery

David Bosanquet, Christopher Wilcox, Rachel Hargest

INTRODUCTION

Randomized controlled trials (RCTs) are important in providing the evidence based on which surgery is practiced. However, many surgical trials are poorly designed or inadequately powered to answer the questions which they propose to address. This chapter details key RCTs undertaken in the field of general surgery between 2015 and 2017 (June). It is not an exhaustive list, but tries to emphasize well-conducted trials, and those with important positive or negative results, which will influence future surgical practice.

GENERAL SURGERY

Surgical teams

The importance of teamwork in surgery cannot be overemphasized. Many of the academic studies of team working issues come from the aviation or business sectors but there is now an emerging field of team working research. One recent publication is of a parallel group cluster randomized trial of the impact of team training on surgical outcomes.[1] Over 22,000 patients were treated by teams from 31 hospitals, randomly assigned to participate in a team training program focused on resource management and checklist utilization (NCT01384474). The primary outcome measure was death or the occurrence of any serious adverse event. Sixteen hospitals received team training, and the event rate fell from 8.8% before training to 5.5% after training (p < 0.0001), while in 15 hospitals that did not receive team training, the event rate fell from 7.9% to 5.4% (p < 0.001). There was therefore no difference between the two trial groups, and it is not possible to conclude that training is necessary but not effective. However, there was a significant fall in event rates across all groups and it may be that the heightened awareness of these issues, along with a changing surgical team culture, may account for these improvements.

Perioperative bridging anticoagulation in patients with atrial fibrillation

In patients, with atrial fibrillation (AF), who require temporary interruption of warfarin treatment for an elective operation or procedure, the need for perioperative bridging anticoagulation remains a subject of debate. The double-blinded, noninferiority "Bridging Anticoagulation in Patients who require Temporary Interruption of Warfarin Therapy for an Elective Invasive Procedure or Surgery" (BRIDGE) trial (NCT00786474) of 1,884 patients investigated rates of arterial thromboembolism and major bleeding, comparing "treatment-dose" low-molecular-weight heparin (LMWH) bridging (Dalteparin) to matching placebo.[2] After 30 days, arterial thromboembolism rates were similar, occurring in 3 of 895 (0.3%) patients in the bridging group and 4 of 918 (0.4%) patients in the placebo group [95% confidence interval (CI) –0.6 to 0.8]. Major bleeding was more than twice as common in the bridging group than the placebo group (3.2% vs 1.3%, p = 0.005), with no fatal events. Rates of minor bleeding were also significantly higher in the bridging group (20.9% vs 12.0%, p < 0.001).

Consistent with a preceding meta-analysis of nonrandomized studies,[3] these data support a strategy of withholding bridging anticoagulation with LMWH in patients with AF who undergo interventional procedures. While data regarding bleeding are relatively strong, current UK practice would still give "prophylactic" LMWH to in-patients with AF who have warfarin discontinued temporarily. Interestingly, there was only a single occurrence of venous thromboembolism (VTE) in this study (in the bridging group). It should also be noted that patients at particularly high-risk of thromboembolism (CHADS2 scores of 5–6) or major bleeding (e.g. neurosurgery) were poorly represented or excluded from the study, respectively. The debate, therefore, remains about how best to manage these patients.

Prevention or treatment of postoperative nausea and vomiting

A significant proportion of patients experience postoperative nausea and vomiting (PONV) and this may have a major impact on patient's comfort, length of stay, and complications including bleeding. There has been a scarcity of well-conducted studies in this field, but two well-conducted trials in this area have recently been reported.

The DREAMS trial (Dexamethasone vs Standard Treatment for Postoperative Nausea and Vomiting in Gastrointestinal Surgery) (ISRCTN21973627) is an RCT of the addition of a single dose of 8 mg intravenous dexamethasone at induction of anesthesia to reduce the incidence of PONV.[4] This UK-based trial randomized 1,250 patients undergoing intestinal surgery to dexamethasone (n = 674) or standard case (n = 676) and the incidence of PONV at 24 hours was 25.5% and 33.0%, respectively in the two groups (p = 0.003 and CI 5–22). Reduction in the need for additional postoperative antiemetics persisted to 72 hours, postoperatively.

The single center, double-blind superiority tPONV trial (NCT01189292) randomized 152 patients undergoing thyroidectomy for benign disease to receive either a single preoperative dose of dexamethasone (8 mg) or placebo.[5] Patients underwent standardized thyroid surgery, during which they received a bilateral superficial cervical plexus block to reduce postoperative pain. After 48 hours, dexamethasone almost halved the incidence of PONV compared to placebo (29% vs 57%, p = 0.001). Furthermore, the severity of PONV was significantly reduced (p = 0.024). Postoperative pain and the incidence of mortality, morbidity, or complications did not differ significantly between groups. There was no reduction in length of stay.

While the PONV rating scale used is not yet validated, it was based on objective symptoms and these results are of clinical significance given that many patients consider PONV to be worse than postoperative pain.

Closure of midline abdominal incisions

Incisional hernias (IHs) are the most common complication following midline laparotomy.[6] Such hernias may significantly reduce quality of life, and often require elective or emergency repair. While many surgeons use the "mass closure" technique, with large bites of tissue to close midline incisions, there are theoretical concerns that the nonfascial tissue involved in these bites will invariably become ischemic, resulting in a greater risk of IHs. The STITCH trial examined the effect of "small bite" suture approach on the incidence of IHs after closure of midline incisions.[7] They undertook a multicenter, double-blinded trial of patients undergoing elective surgery, comparing large bites (1 cm bite every 1 cm, looped 1 PDS) in 248 patients, to small bites (5 mm bite every 5 mm, single ended 2-0 PDS) in 276 patients. 97% of patients completed follow-up with clinical and ultrasound examination, at 1 month and 1 year after surgery.

At one year, 21% of 277 patients in the large bites group had IHs (defined as either clinical or radiological, as per European guidelines) versus 13% of 268 patients in the small bites group (p = 0.022). Time of fascial closure took an average of 4 minutes longer in the small bites groups (14 + 6 vs 10 + 4 minutes). There was no significant difference in postoperative complications, readmissions, hernia size, and pain scores between the groups.

This adds to the growing weight of evidence surrounding small bite midline closure. Key to the technique is the avoidance of muscle or fat in the closure, although it also used smaller needles, so further analysis is necessary to establish whether this may have a confounding effect. Given that prophylactic placement of mesh is gaining popularity, particularly in high-risk groups, optimum midline closure methods are likely to be hotly debated in coming years.

Short-course antimicrobial therapy for complicated intra-abdominal infection

Despite advances in the management of complicated intra-abdominal infection, the appropriate duration of antimicrobial therapy after satisfactory source control remains unclear. The traditional approach has been to continue until evidence of sepsis has subsided, typically over 7–14 days. The "Study to Optimize Peritoneal Infection Therapy" (STOP-IT) trial (NCT00657566) set out to establish whether, following adequate source control, a short-course of antibiotics might offer equivalent outcomes.[8]

Across 23 centers in the United States and Canada, 518 patients (mean age 52.2 + 1) with complicated intra-abdominal infection and adequate source control were randomized to a fixed length short-course group (4 + 1 days of antibiotics), or a control group who received antibiotics until 2 days after the resolution of sepsis (fever, leukocytosis, and ileus) for a maximum of 10 days. Source control included both surgical and radiological interventions. Antibiotic selection was at the discretion of the treating doctor. Groups were well matched at baseline, and the number of patients with appendicitis was limited to encompass a broad range of infections.

Adherence to the protocol was poor (81.8% in the short-course group, 72.7% in the control group). The median duration of antibiotics was halved in the short-course group (4 vs 8 days, respectively, p < 0.001). Both groups had similar rates of complications, including surgical-site infection, recurrent intra-abdominal infection or death (composite outcome rates—21.8% in short-course vs 22.3% in control group). A similar trend was noted on the per protocol analysis. However, it took significantly longer to diagnose surgical-site infection (15.1 + 0.6 vs 8.8 + 0.4 days) and recurrent intra-abdominal infection (15.1 + 0.5 vs 10.8 + 0.4 days) in the control group. There was no difference in rates of extra-abdominal or secondary infection.

These findings suggest that with good source control, a fixed short course of antibiotics can offer similar outcomes to a traditional longer approach that is based on resolution of physiological abnormalities. Longer courses appear to delay the diagnosis of severe complications, rather than preventing them. While the relatively high rate of poor-adherence (18% in short-course group) may have introduced bias, these results should be generalizable across a number of settings.

EMERGENCY SURGERY

Evaluation of patient-controlled analgesia versus routine analgesia in emergency department patients with nontraumatic abdominal pain

While the use of patient-controlled analgesia (PCA) is well-established postoperatively, there is a paucity of evidence regarding its use in the emergency setting. The PAin SoluTions in the Emergency Setting (PASTIES) trial (ISRCTN25343280), undertaken in five English hospitals, compared the use of PCA to routine nurse-titrated analgesia in 200 adult emergency department patients who were eventually admitted to an inpatient ward with moderate to severe nontraumatic abdominal pain.[9] Over the 12-hour study period, the total pain recorded was significantly less in the PCA group than the routine treatment group (mean visual analog scale: 35.3 vs 47.3, p = 0.027). Participants in the PCA group were more than twice as likely to be satisfied with their pain control and received significantly more morphine (mean: 36.1 mg vs 23.6 mg).

This trial lays a weak argument for the use of PCA in these patients. This particular patient group is known to be particularly vulnerable to poor pain management, as they transfer to the ward. However, it could be argued that good nursing care with regular multimodal analgesia is achievable and could have resulted in better pain relief in the control group. Furthermore, guidelines on postoperative analgesia recommend nonopioid multimodal analgesia whenever possible, and an attempt to bring this type of pain relief to the emergency department could be viewed as preferable.

Antibiotic therapy versus appendectomy for the treatment of uncomplicated acute appendicitis

Emergency appendectomy has traditionally been the treatment of choice for acute appendicitis, and evidence to the contrary has been limited by poor study design and restrictive patient selection.[10]

The noninferiority "Appendicitis Acuta" (APPAC) trial (NCT01022567) compared early appendectomy to antibiotic therapy in 530 patients (aged 18–60 years) with computed tomography (CT)-confirmed uncomplicated appendicitis at six finish hospitals.[11] Antibiotic patients received 3 days of intravenous ertapenem, followed by 7 days of oral levofloxacin and metronidazole. Primary outcomes were defined as successful completion of the appendectomy, or discharge from hospital without surgery and no recurrent appendicitis during 1-year follow-up for the two groups.

Of the appendectomy group, 99.6% underwent successful surgery, of which the majority had "open" surgery. Of the antibiotic group, 72.7% were successfully treated and 27.3% underwent appendectomy within 1 year. Intention-to-treat yielded a between group difference of −27% (95% CI −31.6% to ∞, p = 0.89). Of the antibiotic patients who later underwent surgery, 92.9% had appendicitis. There were no significant complications associated with delayed appendectomy. The surgical complication rate was significantly higher for appendectomy patients than antibiotic patients who underwent delayed appendectomy (20.5% vs 7%, p = 0.02), as was the overall complication rate (2.8% vs 20.5%, p < 0.001). The length of hospitalization was significantly shorter in the surgical group (p < 0.001).

The major issue with this trial is the different primary outcomes, which will invariably favor the surgical group as "unsuccessful" appendectomies essentially do not occur. Given the complete difference in treatment options, it could be argued a global measure of health outcome, such as overall quality of life, would be preferable. Another significant factor to consider is that CT imaging was a prerequisite to entry into the study; however, this imaging is frequently not obtained preoperatively in UK practice (especially in men) unless diagnosis is uncertain, nor in resource-poor countries. Given these caveats, nonoperative management was often successful, and delayed appendectomy for failed treatment did not result in any major complications. Patients with CT confirmed appendicitis, for whom there is a reason to try and avoid operative intervention, could reasonably be treated with antibiotics.

UPPER GASTROINTESTINAL SURGERY

Same-admission versus interval cholecystectomy for mild gallstone pancreatitis

Cholecystectomy is typically performed around 6 weeks after discharge from hospital for patients with mild gallstone pancreatitis, if deemed suitable for definitive surgery (rather than endoscopic) treatment.[12] Observational data suggest same-admission cholecystectomy can be safe, yet good quality randomized data are absent. The multicenter PONCHO (pancreatitis of biliary origin—optimal timing of cholecystectomy) RCT of 264 patients from 23 Dutch hospitals compared interval to same-admission cholecystectomy for such patients (ISRCTN72764151).[13] Patients were suitable for randomization, once the C-reactive protein (CRP) was less than 100 mg/L (median 5 days after admission). Cholecystectomy was performed within 3 days of randomization in the "same-admission" arm or at 25–30 days for the "interval" arm. The primary composite endpoint was defined as readmission for gallstone-related complications or mortality within 6 months. The primary endpoint occurred in six (5%) of 128 patients in the "same-admission" group, versus 23 (17%) of 136 patients in the "interval" group (risk ratio 0.28, 95% CI 0.12–0.66; p = 0.002). No difference was seen in the number of major operative complications including bile duct injury/leak (one in each group), length of hospital stay, procedural difficulty or number of conversions.

These findings demonstrate that for mild gallstone pancreatitis, same-admission cholecystectomy was safe and reduced the risk of recurrent gallstone-related complications, compared with interval cholecystectomy. While the study was not powered to detect differences in cholecystectomy-related complications, they were rare and a (probably prohibitively) large RCT would be required to examine this in detail. These results encourage a paradigm shift from semi-elective to acute surgery in these patients; however, the predominant problem with embracing this within the surgical community will most likely be one of financial and time constraints. Unfortunately, total healthcare costs were not evaluated in the study.

Bariatric surgery versus conventional medical treatment for obese patients with type 2 diabetes

Bariatric surgery may be more effective than traditional medical management for obese diabetic patients. Several randomized controlled studies have demonstrated that surgical procedures, which include Roux-en-Y gastric bypass, sleeve gastrectomy, biliopancreatic diversion and gastric banding, achieved better glycemic control than medical therapy or lifestyle advice alone. These trials were, however, limited by their short follow-up (1–3 years) and longer-term data is required to fully appreciate the effects of surgical intervention.

Mingrone et al. equally randomized 60 obese patients (aged 30–60 years) with history of diabetes of at least 5 years, to receive medical treatment, gastric bypass or biliopancreatic diversion at a single center in Italy (NCT00888836).[14] The primary outcome was remission of diabetes, defined as a fasting glucose concentration of less than 5.6 and hemoglobin A1C (HbA1C) concentration less than 6.5% without pharmacological treatment for at least 1 year. After 5 years, 53 patients were available for follow up. None of the 15 medical patients achieved remission, versus half of the 38 surgical patients (37% and 63% of the gastric bypass and biliopancreatic diversion groups, respectively, p = 0.007). Surgery was associated with lower plasma lipids, cardiovascular risk, and medication use, a greater quality of life, and was undertaken with minimal surgical morbidity and no early or late mortality.

This study adds to the growing consensus that surgical treatment is more effective than medication alone for obese diabetics. While this study has achieved a longer follow-up than other comparative studies, the sample size is noticeably small. Furthermore, the primary endpoint of diabetes remission favors surgical treatment by definition, as nonsurgical diabetic remission is a rare occurrence, particularly in those who have had the disease for at least 5 years. For long-term follow-up, easily comparable outcome, such as mortality, quality of life, and other standard markers of health are probably of greater value in deciding on best treatment options for patients. However, despite shortcomings in methodology and outcome reporting, surgical intervention for type 2 diabetes is most likely of significant long-term value, and future studies should look at identifying which patients benefit most from surgery.

COLORECTAL SURGERY

Laparoscopic peritoneal lavage versus sigmoidectomy for patients with perforated diverticulitis

In recent years, laparoscopic peritoneal lavage has emerged as a potential alternative to sigmoidectomy in patients with purulent peritonitis secondary to perforated diverticulitis. The LADIES trial (NCT01317485) is a multicenter parallel-armed RCT evaluating surgical management of perforated diverticulitis with either nonfeculent (purulent) peritonitis (the LOLA group) or fecal peritonitis (DIVA group). The LOLA trial enrolled 90 patients (mean age—63 years) across 30 European hospitals, assigned, after laparoscopic confirmed purulent peritonitis due to perforated diverticulitis, to either laparoscopic lavage or sigmoidectomy (with or without primary anastomosis).[15] The primary outcome comprised a composite endpoint of mortality or major morbidity at 12 months. This superiority trial planned to enroll 264 patients, with an expected primary outcome occurring in 10% and 25% of patients in the lavage and sigmoidectomy arms, respectively. It was stopped early due to an increased in-hospital primary outcome event rate in the lavage group compared to the sigmoidectomy group (39% vs 19%; p = 0.0427) of which the majority were surgical reinterventions. After 12 months, there was no significant difference in major morbidity, mortality, or postoperative quality of life.

However, laparoscopic lavage for purulent diverticulitis would be expected to require a greater percentage of reinterventions compared to definitive sigmoidectomy. Therefore by including these reinterventions as a primary outcome, an increase in early events in the lavage group could have been anticipated. However by 12 months, the incidence of primary outcome events was almost identical between groups [67% (lavage) vs 60%]. A superiority or even noninferiority trial based on these figures would have been too large to be feasible. However, while laparoscopy lavage as a first-line treatment appears from these data to require more early interventions; generally, this technique is successful in managing the disease process. Unfortunately, the stoma rate in each cohort was not reported, as this is being examined as part of the DIVA arm of the LADIES trial.

In the absence of any other randomized data, it is difficult to support the routine use of diagnostic lavage for these cases. Historically, the gold standard remains sigmoidectomy, and nonspecialists should consider this standard surgical management. Proponents of laparoscopic lavage may use this data to support this as an appropriate approach, so long as patients are well consented and informed about the high chance of requiring future intervention.

Percutaneous tibial nerve stimulation versus sham electrical stimulation for the treatment of fecal incontinence in adults

Percutaneous tibial nerve stimulation (PTNS) is a novel outpatient therapy for fecal incontinence, which has emerged as a potential alternative to sacral nerve stimulation. The double-blind CONFIDeNT (CONtrol of Faecal Incontinence using Distal NeuromodulaTion) trial (ISRCTN 88559475) was the first to compare the short-term efficacy of PTNS against sham electrical stimulation, involving 227 adults for whom conservative management had failed, across 17 UK hospitals.[16] Therapy was delivered by certified practitioners, for 30 minutes weekly over 12 weeks, and outcomes were assessed using patients' bowel diaries, and validated incontinence and quality-of-life scores.

In contrast to previous data based predominantly on case series, PTNS did not confer a significant treatment response, based on the primary endpoint of more than or equal to 50% reduction in the number of episodes of fecal incontinence per week (38% vs 31% in the sham group, p = 0.396). Furthermore, there were no significant differences in incontinence scores or quality-of-life measures. PTNS did result in a significant reduction in mean total episodes of fecal incontinence per week (−2.26, p = 0.02) and urge incontinence (−1.46 p = 0.02); however, these differences were small and arguably of little clinical significance.

There is ongoing debate regarding what represents the optimum measure for fecal incontinence. The primary endpoint used in this trial represents an outcome used in the majority of pivotal incontinence studies and allows comparisons to be drawn between various treatment modalities. Furthermore, there is a lack of consensus regarding what entails "failed" conservative therapy and the patients recruited for this trial were not formally standardized. Importantly, while CONFIDeNT may only weakly support the use PTNS in this setting, it stresses the need for further well-designed trials, which explore its efficacy long term, and potential use within various subgroups of patients.

Crohn's disease management after intestinal resection

Most patients with Crohn's disease will end up undergoing intestinal resection, and unfortunately the majority of these will require further surgery to treat recurrence. The treat-to-target POCER (postoperative Crohn's endoscopic recurrence) trial (NCT00989560) was the first to assess strategies to reduce disease recurrence in postoperative Crohn's patients.[17]

Over two years, 174 consecutive patients from 17 centers in Australia and New Zealand were randomized in a 2:1 ratio to receive active or standard care (with or without a colonoscopy at 6 months, respectively). Patients received 3 months of metronidazole therapy, and those at high-risk of recurrence also received a thiopurine (or adalimumab if they were intolerant). For the active group, in cases of endoscopic recurrence at 6 months, patients were stepped-up to thiopurine, fortnightly adalimumab with thiopurine, or weekly adalimumab.

Endoscopic recurrence at 18 months was less common in the active care group (49%) than the standard care group (67%), p = 0.03. Furthermore, complete mucosal normality was maintained in more of the active care group (22%) than the standard care group (8%), p = 0.03. The incidence and type of adverse events did not differ significantly between the groups. Of 122 active care patients, 47 (39%) with endoscopic recurrence stepped up treatment at 6 months. Of these 47, 38% were brought into remission at 1 year. Despite effective drug therapy, smoking doubled the risk of endoscopic recurrence (odds ratio 2:4, 95% CI 1.2–4.8, p = 0.02).

Early colonoscopy after surgery is rarely performed in clinical practice. However, this trial demonstrated that a structured approach using 6-month colonoscopy and treatment step-up for selected patients with recurrence, confers effective disease control in most patients, and is significantly better than optimum drug therapy alone. Importantly, it should be noted that early endoscopic remission did not guarantee maintenance of remission, and continued monitoring of these patients is warranted.

Laparoscopic versus open surgery for rectal cancer

Laparoscopic surgery is well established within the field of colonic surgery but there is less evidence from large trials to support its use in rectal cancer. Three important trials reported outcomes of laparoscopic rectal cancer. The first is the International noninferiority COLOR II trial (NCT00297791), which recruited 1,044 patients with primary rectal adenocarcinoma (within 15 cm from the anal verge), across 30 hospitals.[18] Patient was randomized to either laparoscopic or open surgery (2:1 ratio) and analyzed by intention-to-treat. Baseline characteristics and the rate of neoadjuvant chemotherapy use were similar for both groups.

After 3 years, laparoscopic surgery was associated with similar rates of locoregional recurrence (both 5%, 95% CI −2.6 to 2.6). There was also no difference in rates of disease-free survival (74.8% vs 70.8%, 95% CI −1.9 to 9.9) and overall survival (86.7% vs 83.6%, 95% CI −1.6 to 7.8), although for stage III cancer, disease-free survival was greater after laparoscopic surgery (64.9% vs 52% difference, 95% CI 2.2 to 23.6). Furthermore, while laparoscopic surgery took longer (240 vs 188 minutes, p < 0.0001), bowel function returned sooner (2 vs 3 days, p < 0.0001) and hospital stay was shorter (8 vs 9 days, p = 0.036).[19] There were no significant differences in procedure-related complications, morbidity, or mortality.

In contrast, two further studies published in 2015 used essentially equivalent methods to examine laparoscopic and open surgery in terms of gross pathologic and histological evaluation of the excised specimen. Fleshman et al. randomized 462 patients in America with stage II or III rectal cancer (ACOSOGG Z6051) (NCT00726622), while the similar Australasian trial (ALaCaRT) (ACTRN1260900066325) randomized 475 patients with T1-T3 rectal tumors.[20,21] A successful resection was defined as one with a composite of circumferential radial margin greater than 1 mm, distal margin without tumor, and completeness of total mesorectal excision. Both studies found laparoscopic surgery was inferior to open surgery, with regards to successful resection. What is noticeable about these results is that they report a surrogate outcome (histological assessment), in the absence of clinically meaningful outcomes.

There were some significant differences between these three studies. The distribution of cancer location, the proportion of patients with advanced disease and the proportion receiving neoadjuvant chemotherapy (100% in ACOSOG Z6051 vs 59% in COLOR II) differed widely, meaning that harmonizing these three trials is difficult. Surgical practice is unlikely to swing away from laparoscopic rectal surgery in the absence of patient-specific outcomes. Furthermore, various groups appear to have improved outcome with laparoscopic surgery. In COLOR II, cancer in the lower third of the rectum was associated with a lower rate of involved circumferential resection margin and locoregional recurrence rate following laparoscopic surgery versus open surgery (4.4% vs 11.7%). In such narrow spaces, laparoscopy can improve the operative field-of-view and may actually improve survival.

Robotic versus laparoscopic surgery for rectal cancer

Robotic surgery has been taken up enthusiastically by surgeons for a variety of procedures. However, there is little evidence for its benefits in terms of measurable outcomes. The International multicentre RObotic versus LAparoscopic Resection for Rectal Cancer (ROLARR) trial (ISRCTN 80500123) of robotic versus laparoscopic surgery for rectal cancer.[22] The primary outcome measure was conversion to open surgery. Over 470 patients were randomized in this study and were followed up for up to 2 years. There was no significant difference in conversion rates to open surgery. Secondary endpoints included CRM (circumferential margin) positivity rates, intraoperative and postoperative complication rates, pathological plane of resection, urinary and sexual dysfunction, and 30-day mortality also showed no significant difference between groups. In conclusion, the ROLARR trial has shown no benefit for robotic surgery over laparoscopic surgery for rectal cancer.

Screening for colorectal cancer

The UK Flexible Sigmoidoscopy Screening Trial (ISRCTN, number 28352761), which was originally carried out between 1994 and 1999 published its long-term outcomes recently.[23] It concluded that a single flexible sigmoidoscopy (between the ages of 55-64) continues to provide substantial protection from colorectal cancer diagnosis and death, with protection lasting at least 17 years. Over 170,000 individuals were included in the trial and had originally been randomized (1:2) to either intervention or control groups. The intervention group was invited for flexible sigmoidoscopy screening. Details of the trial and its shorter term outcomes have already been published.[24] Colorectal cancer was diagnosed in 1230/57098 (2.15%) individuals in the intervention group and 3253/112 936 (2.88%) in the control group. Over the following 17 years, deaths from colorectal cancer occurred in 353 individuals in the intervention group versus 996 individuals in the control group. Intention-to-treat analyses showed that colorectal cancer incidence was reduced by 26% [heart rate (HR) 0•74 (95% CI 0.70–0.80); $p < 0.0001$] and colorectal cancer mortality was reduced by 30% [0.70 (0.62–0.79); $p < 0.0001$] in the intervention group versus the control group. In per-protocol analyses, adjusted for noncompliance, colorectal cancer incidence, and mortality were 35% [HR 0.65 (95% CI 0.59–0.71)] and 41% [0.59 (0.49–0.70)] lower in the screened group. These results appear to make a convincing argument for the use of flexible sigmoidoscopy for colorectal cancer screening. However, there are several confounding factors including the effect of compliance versus noncompliance with screening. Although randomization was performed in blocks to control for geography and various types of general practice, individuals who take up the offer of screening are likely to be those who take greater care of their health generally and therefore may adopt healthier diets, activities or be less likely to smoke, drink excessive alcohol, or undertake other unhealthy pursuits.

BREAST SURGERY

Cavity shave margins in breast cancer

Among women undergoing wide local excision (WLE) for breast cancer, the use of cavity shave margins may reduce the rate of positive margins (for tumor cells). The presence of a positive margin most often results in subsequent re-excision. Chagpar et al. (2015) conducted the first RCT (NCT01452399) comparing the routine use of cavity margin shave, with standard practice, and recruited 235 women (mean age 61 years) with biopsy-confirmed breast cancer (stages 0–III) who were undoing WLE.[25] After standard WLE, patients were randomized intraoperatively (1:1) to either a further cavity shave group, or a no-shave group. Groups were well-matched, received similar neoadjuvant chemotherapy (both 3%) and had a similar rate of positive margins before randomization (36% vs 35%, p = 0.69), which did not vary according to surgeon, age, or tumor size.

Cavity shaving significantly reduced the rate of positive margins (19% vs 34%, p = 0.01) and halved the rate of reoperation (10% vs 21%, p = 0.02), without differences in complications or patients' perception of cosmetic outcomes. The median total volume of tissue excised was significantly larger for shave patients (115.1 cm^3 vs 74.2 cm^3, p < 0.001). These findings reflect those reported by previous retrospective studies. Systematic cavity shaves may be appropriate for those undergoing WLE.

Prevention of alopecia during chemotherapy for breast cancer

An interesting multicenter trial from USA, randomized women undergoing chemotherapy for stage I–III breast cancer to receive scalp cooling or control. The SCALP study (NCT01986140) carried out a single-blinded randomized trial using a commercial scalp cooling device (Paxman, UK) during chemotherapy with taxane- or anthracycline-based chemotherapy.[26] Measurement of hair loss was performed according to the 4 grade Common Terminology Criteria for Adverse Events version 4.0 scale where Grade 0 = no hair loss and Grade 4 = complete alopecia. The primary endpoint was hair loss of less than 50% and not requiring a wig. There was significant benefit in the group receiving scalp cooling where 50.5% preserved at least 50% of their hair compared to none in the noncooled group (p = 0.0061).

Medical treatment of breast cancer

The majority of clinical trials in the field of breast cancer treatment are concerned with chemotherapy, radiotherapy, and hormonal treatments. It would not be possible to comment on all of these trials in this chapter but the important recent publications are listed in **Table 14.1**.

Table 14.1: Clinical trials relating to medical treatment of breast cancer (2015–2017).[27-35]

Trial	Summary	Outcome	Reference	Registration
HERA	Long-term (11 years) outcome of trastuzumab in early HER2+ BC	Trastuzumab for 1 year improved DFS and OS, but there was no benefit for the 2nd year	Cameron et al.	NCT00045032
CREATE-X	Addition of capecitabine after neoadjuvant chemotherapy for residual HER-BC	Capecitabine significantly improved 5-year DFS and OS	Masuda et al.	UMIN000000843
PANTHER	Tailored dose versus standard cycle adjuvant chemotherapy for women with early BC	Tailored dose chemotherapy did not improve DFS or OS compare with standard regimes	Foukakis et al.	NCT00798070; ISRCTN39017665
MA.17R MA.17	Extending AI therapy to 10 years	Extending AI to 10 years produced significantly less CBC and improved DFS, but no significant difference in OS	Goss et al.	NCT00003140 NCT00754845
I-SPY 2	Addition of neratinib versus standard NACT for appropriate genetic subtypes of BC	Addition of neratinib increased PCR rates compared to standard NECT	Park et al.	NCT01042379
I-SPY 2	Addition of Veliparib–Carboplatin for HER-BC	Addition of Veliparib–Carboplatin improved PCR rates in the triple negative BCs	Rugo et al.	NCT01042379
IBIS II DCIS	Adjuvant anastrozole versus tamoxifen in postmenopausal women with hormone receptor positive DCIS	There was NSD in LRR or CBC in the two groups	Forbes et al.	ISRCTN37546358
NSABP B-35	Adjuvant anastrozole versus tamoxifen in postmenopausal women with hormone receptor positive DCIS	Anastrozole increased the BC-free interval in women < 60 years	Margolese et al.	NCT00053898
Interstitial brachy-therapy alone versus external beam radiation therapy after breast conserving surgery for low risk invasive carcinoma and low-risk duct carcinoma in situ (DCIS) of the female breast	WBI versus APBI after BCS in women with early BC	There was NSD in the rates of LRR at 5 years	Strnad et al.	NCT00402519

(AI: Aromatase inhibitor; APBI: Accelerated partial breast irradiation; BC: Breast cancer; BCS: Breast-conserving surgery; CBC: Contralateral breast cancer; DFS: Disease-free survival; HER: Herceptin receptor; LRR: Locoregional recurrence; NACT: Neoadjuvant chemotherapy; NSD: No significant difference; OS: Overall survival; PCR: Pathological complete response; ABI: Whole breast irradiation).

VASCULAR SURGERY

Long-term outcomes after stenting versus endarterectomy for treatment of symptomatic carotid stenosis

Carotid endarterectomy (CEA) is commonly performed to lower the risk of stroke in patients with symptomatic atherosclerotic stenosis of the internal carotid artery. The Internal Carotid Stenting Study (ISRCTN25337470) was a large international trial of 1,713 patients across 50 centers, which set out to investigate carotid stenting as a possible alternative treatment.[36] Participants, aged over 40 years, all had internal carotid arterial stenoses of greater than 50%.

At a median follow-up of 4.2 years, the number (52 of stented patients vs 49 CEA patients) and cumulative 5-year risk (6.4% vs 6.5%) of fatal or disabling strokes did not differ significantly between groups (p = 0.77). The incidence of any stroke type was more frequent in the stenting group (119 vs 72, p = 0.0003). This difference was mainly attributable to the number of nondisabling strokes (73 vs 27), and no difference in short- or long-term functional outcomes, or quality of life, was seen between groups. This finding should be weighed against the increased risk of procedural myocardial infarction, cranial nerve palsy, and access-site hematoma following carotid endarterectomy, which has been demonstrated in previous RCTs.[37]

The ACT 1 randomized trial (NCT00106938) (of stenting vs surgery for asymptomatic carotid artery stenosis was stopped after 14,453 patients were randomized due to slow enrolment. At termination the risk of death, stroke or myocardial infarction at 30 days or ipsilateral stroke within 1 year was 3.8% for stenting and 3.4% for surgery (p = 0.01).[38]

However, this paper, along with other RCTs, has shown an increased risk of stroke with stenting compared to open surgery. While stenting has been embraced in certain areas of the USA, it is likely that within the UK stenting will only be available in a few centers of excellence, and its use restricted to complex cases where open surgery would be dangerous or difficult.

Endovascular versus open repair strategy for ruptured abdominal aortic aneurysms

Despite improvements in operative technique, ruptured abdominal aortic aneurysm (rAAA) is often fatal and operative mortality remains high. The less invasive endovascular aneurysm repair (EVAR) has become a well-established treatment modality for elective procedures, but emergency EVAR is not available in all centers and the majority of rAAA cases globally undergo open repair.

Previous RCTs have demonstrated no survival benefit for the endovascular strategy at 30 days.[39,40]

A more recent publication from the IMPROVE trial group reported long-term outcomes.[41] After 1 year, all-cause mortality for "endovascular first" strategy (41.1%) was similar to open repair (45.1%, odds ratio 0.85; 95% CI 0.62, 1.17, p = 0.325), as were reintervention rates. An endovascular first strategy was associated with reduced hospital stay (17 vs 26 days, p < 0.001), reduced cost-effective and better quality of life.

While the results could be interpreted as surprising, the IMPROVE trial (ISRCTN 48334791) has shown that mortality is directly related to AAA neck length. The longer the neck, the more likely EVAR is possible, and when analyzed by treatment actually received, patients who received EVAR did considerably better than those undergoing open repair. However, even within the open group, the longer the neck length the better the outcomes. Anatomical suitability is therefore a predictor of improved outcomes of a ruptured AAA, irrespective of the actual treatment modality received.

Paclitaxel-coated balloons for femoropopliteal artery disease

While treatment with percutaneous transluminal angioplasty may initially restore or improve lower limb blood flow for patients with femoropopliteal artery disease, many patients suffer from vessel recoil, restenosis, and neointimal hyperplasia within 1 year. Drug-coated angioplasty balloons, which deliver antiproliferative agents directly to the artery, might reduce restenosis and improve long-term vessel patency.

The international, single-blinded LEVANT 2 trial randomized 476 patients at 54 sites to either a paclitaxel-coated, or conventional angioplasty balloon (control) group, in a 2:1 ratio.[42] Patients had moderate or severe claudication, or rest pain (Rutherford stage two to four) and a significant a femoropopliteal atherosclerotic lesion.

After one year, the paclitaxel-coated group had a significantly higher rate of primary patency (65.2% vs 52.6%, p = 0.02), as assessed by blinded analysis of duplex ultrasonography. Both techniques resulted in similar improvement of functional outcomes and quality of life. Rates of death (2.4 vs 2.8%), amputation (0.3% vs 0%), and thrombosis requiring reintervention (0.4% vs 0.7%) were similar for drug-coated and standard groups, respectively.

While the results are supportive of paclitaxel-coated balloons, there are a number of points which should be highlighted. Firstly, this is an industry-sponsored study. Secondly, over 90% of all patients were claudicants. Treatment of this group is predominantly with exercise, smoking cessation, and "best medical therapy". Few UK patients with claudication would receive angioplasty, and fewer still would be offered therapies other than basic angioplasty in the absence of critical limb ischemia. Thirdly, a cost analysis is lacking; it may be that the marginal patency improvement is offset by a substantial cost, which makes these drug-eluting balloons nonfinancially viable. Fourthly, vessel patency is a surrogate marker of clinical success. Symptomatic improvement, or in the context of tissue loss, and wound healing are more clinically important outcomes.

CONCLUSION

This chapter has highlighted a tiny minority of the important clinical trials in surgery of the last 2 years. Time and space does not permit a more extensive analysis. However, we hope that this selection will stimulate readers to explore the literature of their branch of surgery for themselves, in order to keep up-to-date and hence offer their own patients the best evidence-based surgical care.

REFERENCES

1. Duclos A, Peix JL, Piriou V, et al. Cluster randomized trial to evaluate the impact of team training on surgical outcomes. Br J Surg. 2016;103(13):1804-14.
2. Douketis JD, Spyropoulos AC, Kaatz S, et al; BRIDGE Investigators. Perioperative Bridging Anticoagulation in Patients with Atrial Fibrillation. N Engl J Med. 2015;373(9):823-33.
3. Siegal D, Yudin J, Kaatz S, et al. Periprocedural heparin bridging in patients receiving vitamin K antagonists: systematic review and meta-analysis of bleeding and thromboembolic rates. Circulation. 2012;126(13): 1630-9.

4. DREAMS Trial Collaborators and West Midlands Research Collaborative. Dexamethasone versus standard treatment for postoperative nausea and vomiting in gastrointestinal surgery: randomised controlled trial (DREAMS Trial). BMJ. 2017;357:j1455.
5. Tarantino I, Warschkow R, Beutner U, et al. Efficacy of a single preoperative dexamethasone dose to prevent nausea and vomiting after thyroidectomy (the tPONV Study): a randomized, double-blind, placebo-controlled clinical trial. Ann Surg. 2015;262(6):934-40.
6. Fink C, Baumann P, Wente MN, et al. Incisional hernia rate 3 years after midline laparotomy. Br J Surg. 2014;101(2):51-4.
7. Deerenberg EB, Harlaar JJ, Steyerberg EW, et al. Small bites versus large bites for closure of abdominal midline incisions (STITCH): a double-blind, multicentre, randomised controlled trial. Lancet. 2015;386(10000): 1254-60.
8. Sawyer RG, Claridge JA, Nathens AB, et al. Trial of short-course antimicrobial therapy for intraabdominal infection. N Eng J Med. 2015;372(21):1996-2005.
9. Smith JE, Rockett M, Creanor S, et al. PAin SoluTions In the Emergency Setting (PASTIES)—patient controlled analgesia versus routine care in emergency department patients with non-traumatic abdominal pain: randomised trial. BMJ. 2015;350:h2988.
10. Wilms IM, de Hoog DE, de Visser DC, et al. Appendectomy versus antibiotic treatment for acute appendicitis. Cochrane Database Syst Rev. 2011;11:Cd008359.
11. Salminen P, Paajanen H, Rautio T, et al. Antibiotic therapy vs appendectomy for treatment of uncomplicated acute appendicitis: the APPAC randomized clinical trial. JAMA. 313(23):2340-8.
12. Besselink M vSH, Freeman M, Gardner T, et al. IAP/APA evidence-based guidelines for the management of acute pancreatitis. Pancreatology. 2013;13(4 Suppl 2):e1-15.
13. Da Costa DW, Bouwense SA, Schepers NJ, et al. Same-admission versus interval cholecystectomy for mild gallstone pancreatitis (PONCHO): a multicentre randomised controlled trial. Lancet. 2015;386(10000): 1261-8.
14. Mingrone G, Panunzi S, De Gaetano A, et al. Bariatric–metabolic surgery versus conventional medical treatment in obese patients with type 2 diabetes: 5-year follow-up of an open-label, single-centre, randomised controlled trial. Lancet. 2015;386(9997):964-73.
15. Vennix S, Musters GD, Mulder IM, et al. Laparoscopic peritoneal lavage or sigmoidectomy for perforated diverticulitis with purulent peritonitis: a multicentre, parallel-group, randomised, open-label trial. The Lancet. 2015;386(10000):1269-77.
16. Knowles CH, Horrocks EJ, Bremner SA, et al. Percutaneous tibial nerve stimulation versus sham electrical stimulation for the treatment of faecal incontinence in adults (CONFIDeNT): a double-blind, multicentre, pragmatic, parallel-group, randomised controlled trial. Lancet. 2015;386(10004):1640-8.
17. De Cruz P, Kamm MA, Hamilton AL, et al. Crohn's disease management after intestinal resection: a randomised trial. Lancet. 2015;385(9976):1406-17.
18. Bonjer HJ, Deijen CL, Abis GA, et al. A Randomized trial of laparoscopic versus open surgery for rectal cancer. N Engl J Med. 2015;372(14):1324-32.
19. Van der Pas MH, Haglind E, Cuesta MA, et al. Laparoscopic versus open surgery for rectal cancer (COLOR II): short-term outcomes of a randomised, phase 3 trial. Lancet Oncol. 2015;14(3):210-8.
20. Fleshman J, Branda M, Sargent DJ, et al. Effect of laparoscopic-assisted resection vs open resection of stage ii or iii rectal cancer on pathologic outcomes: The ACOSOGG Z6051 randomized clinical trial. JAMA. 2015;314(13):1346-55.
21. Stevenson AR, Solonon MJ, Lumley JW, et al. Effect of laparoscopic-assisted resection vs open resection on pathological outcomes in rectal cancer: the ALaCaRT randomized clinical trial. JAMA. 2015;314(13): 1356-63.
22. Jayne D, Pigazzi A, Marshall H, et al. Effect of robotic-assisted vs conventional laparoscopic surgery on risk of conversion to open laparotomy among patients undergoing resection for rectal cancer: the ROLARR randomized clinical trial. JAMA. 2017;318(16):1569-80.
23. Atkin W, Wooldrage K, Parkin DM, et al. Long term effects of once-only flexible sigmoidoscopy screening after 17 years of follow-up: the UK Flexible Sigmoidoscopy Screening randomised controlled trial. Lancet. 2017;389(10076):1299-311.
24. Atkin WS, Edwards R, Kralj-Hans I, et al; UK Flexible Sigmoidoscopy Trial Investigators. Once-only flexible sigmoidoscopy screening in prevention of colorectal cancer: a multicentre randomised controlled trial. Lancet. 2010;375(9726):1624-33.
25. Chagpar AB, Killelea BK, Tsangaris TN, et al. A randomized, controlled trial of cavity shave margins in breast cancer. N Engl J Med. 2015;373(6):503-10.

26. Nangia J, Wang T, Osborne C, et al. Effect of a scalp cooling device on alopecia in women undergoing chemotherapy for breast cancer: the SCALP randomized clinical trial. JAMA. 2017;317(6):596-605.
27. Cameron D, Piccart-Gebhart MJ, Gelber RD, et al. 11 years' follow-up of trastuzumab after adjuvant chemotherapy in HER2-positive early breast cancer: final analysis of the HERceptin Adjuvant (HERA) trial. Lancet. 2017;389(10075):1195-205.
28. Masuda N, Lee SJ, Ohtani S, et al. Adjuvant capecitabine for breast cancer after preoperative chemotherapy. N Engl J Med. 2017;376(22):2147-59.
29. Foukakis T, von Minckwitz G, Bengtsson NO, et al. Effect of tailored dose-dense chemotherapy vs standard 3-weekly adjuvant chemotherapy on recurrence-free survival among women with high-risk early breast cancer: a randomized clinical trial. JAMA. 2016;316(18):1888-96.
30. Goss PE, Ingle JN, Pritchard KI, et al. Extending aromatase-inhibitor adjuvant therapy to 10 Years. N Engl J Med. 2016;375(3):209-19.
31. Park JW, Liu MC, Yee D, et al. Adaptive randomization of neratinib in early breast cancer. N Engl J Med. 2016;375(1):11-22.
32. Rugo HS, Olopade OI, DeMichele A, et al. Adaptive randomization of veliparib-carboplatin treatment in breast cancer. N Engl J Med. 2016;375(1):23-34.
33. Forbes JF, Sestak I, Howell A, et al. Anastrozole versus tamoxifen for the prevention of locoregional and contralateral breast cancer in postmenopausal women with locally excised ductal carcinoma in situ (IBIS-II DCIS): a double-blind, randomised controlled trial. Lancet. 2016;387(10021):866-73.
34. Margolese RG, Cecchini RS, Julian TB, et al. Anastrozole versus tamoxifen in postmenopausal women with ductal carcinoma in situ undergoing lumpectomy plus radiotherapy (NSABP B-35): a randomised, double-blind, phase 3 clinical trial. Lancet. 2016;387(10021):849-56.
35. Strnad V, Ott OJ, Hildebrandt G, et al. 5-year results of accelerated partial breast irradiation using sole interstitial multicatheter brachytherapy versus whole-breast irradiation with boost after breast-conserving surgery for low-risk invasive and in-situ carcinoma of the female breast: a randomised, phase 3, non-inferiority trial. Lancet. 2016;387(10015):229-38.
36. Bonati LH, Dobson J, Featherstone RL, et al. Long-term outcomes after stenting versus endarterectomy for treatment of symptomatic carotid stenosis: the International Carotid Stenting Study (ICSS) randomised trial. Lancet. 2015;385(9967):529-38.
37. Bonati LH, Lyrer P, Ederle J, et al. Percutaneous transluminal balloon angioplasty and stenting for carotid artery stenosis. 2015 Cochrane Database Syst Rev. 2012;(9):Cd000515.
38. Rosenfield K, Matsumura JS, Chaturvedi S, et al. Randomized trial of stent versus surgery for asymptomatic carotid stenosis. N Engl J Med. 2016;374(11):1011-20.
39. Reimerink JJ, Hoornweg LL, Vahl AC, et al. Endovascular repair versus open repair of ruptured abdominal aortic aneurysms: a multicenter randomized controlled trial. Ann Surg. 2013;258(2):248-56.
40. IMPROVE Trial Investigators, Powell JT, Sweeting MJ, et al. Endovascular or open repair strategy for ruptured abdominal aortic aneurysm: 30 day outcomes from IMPROVE randomised trial. BMJ. 2014;348:f7661.
41. IMPROVE Trial Investigators. Endovascular strategy or open repair for ruptured abdominal aortic aneurysm: one-year outcomes from the IMPROVE randomized trial. Eur Heart J. 2015;36(31):2061-9.
42. Rosenfield K, Jaff MR, White CJ, et al. Trial of a paclitaxel-coated balloon for femoropopliteal artery disease. N Engl J Med. 2015;373(2):145-53.

Index

Page numbers followed by *f* refer to figure, *fc* refer to flowchart, and *t* refer to table.

A

Abdominal cavity 69
Abdominal esophagus 71
Abdominal incisions, closure of midline 158
Abdominoperineal resection 85, 98
Abscesses in
 liver 97
 pharynx 10
Accelerated partial breast irradiation 167
Acid-fast bacilli 95, 96, 99
Acrylonitrile butadiene styrene 145
Actinomycosis 97
Adjuvant anastrozole 167
Adjuvant cisplatin 86
Adjuvant radiotherapy 37
Aerodigestive structures 69
Agarose 146
Alginate 146
Allegations 22
Alopecia during chemotherapy for breast cancer, prevention of 166
American Association for the Surgery of Trauma Organ Injury Scale
 lacerations–duodenum 70, 76*t*
 lacerations–esophagus 70*t*
 lacerations–stomach 75*t*
American Joint Committee on Cancer 61
Aminosalicylates 105
Amoebiasis 97
Anal cancer
 cases of 85
 chemoradiation for 92
 cross-sectional CT imaging to 88*f*
 incidence rate of 85
 radiation for 86
 role of chemoradiotherapy in the treatment of 86
 role of surgery in the treatment of 85
 trials: targeted agents/immunotherapy in combination with radiation 91
Anal fissure 95
Anal ulceration 95
Aneurysm 134
Anomalous first rib 134
Anoperineal tuberculosis 94
Anorectal and perineal manifestations of tuberculosis
 clinical presentation and manifestations 95
 diagnosis 95
 pathogenesis 94
 treatment 98
Anorectal sepsis 95
Anorectal tuberculosis 94
Antacids 106
Antibiotic therapy 160
Antimicrobial
 therapy for complicated intra-abdominal infection 159
 treatment 9
Antiretroviral therapy 98
Anti-TNF drugs 105
Antitubercular therapy 98
Antitumor responses 92
Aphthous ulcers 97
Apology 22
Appendectomy 160
 group 160
Appendicitis, acute, treatment of uncomplicated 160
Appendix 94
Aromatase inhibitor 167
Arterial thoracic outlet syndrome 134
 clinical presentation and diagnosis 134
 management 136
Association for Breast Surgery, guidelines 50
Associative phase of Fitts and Posner's model 28
Atrial fibrillation 157
Atypical hyperplasia, forms of 46
Atypical lobular hyperplasia 45
Autonomous 27
Azygos vein, division of 73

B

Bacillus Calmette–Guérin 99
Bariatric surgery 162
Bioinks 146
BioVision 40
Blindness to ordinary experience 29
Bolam versus Friern Hospital Management Committee, 1957 18
Bolitho versus City and Hackney Health Authority, 1997 18
Bones and joints 94
Boot camps 28
Bowel symptoms, questionnaire scores for 90
Brachial plexus 127
 injuries 128
Brachytherapy 90
Bragg peak 91
Breast cancer 167
 bilateral 46
 cavity shave margins in 166

clinical trials relating to medical treatment of 167t
contralateral 46
medical treatment of 166
reported 37
surgery, assessment of margins in 37
Breast surgery 166
Breast-conserving surgery 167
Breast-screening programs, widespread use of 38
Buccal cavity 69
Budesonide 105
Bulky symptomatic tumors, presence of 86

C

Cancer of head and neck 55
Cancer, risk of developing 85
Carboplatin 92
Cardiac cycle 30
    diastole 30
    systole 30
Cardiac transplantation 148
Cardiothoracic surgery 148
Carotid endarterectomy 168
Carpal tunnel syndrome 128
Catastrophic consequences 75
Cavity shave 40
CDH1 46
Central necrosis, areas of 58
Central nervous systems 94
Cerenkov luminescence imaging 41
Cervical disk disease 128
Cervical esophageal fistulas 74
Cervical esophagus 70, 72
    penetrating injuries of 72
Cervical lymph node 55
    diagnostic dilemma in clinically 56
    evaluation of 56
    histopathological examination of 55
    metastases evolution of surgery for 57
    surgical staging of 56
Cervical precancerous lesions 85
Cervical rib 126, 134
    presence of 134
Cervical spine reconstruction 148
Cesarean section 107
Chemical analysis 41
Chemotherapy
    backbone treatment 92
    cycles of 86
Chest 69, 73
Cholecystectomy 161
Cholestyramine 106
Chromosomal gains (1q) 49
Chronic active disease 103
Cisplatin/5-FU 91, 92
Civil Court rules 22
Claimant's expert report 16

Claimant's solicitor 16
Claims made 21
Clearedge 40, 41
Clinical negligence scheme for trusts 13
Clinical target volume 88
Clostridium perfringens 5, 116
Clostridium septicum 5
Clostridium sordellii 5
Codeine 106
Cognitive training 32
Collagen 146
Colon, ascending 94
Colonic skip lesions 97
Colonoscopy after surgery 164
Colorectal cancer 116
    screening for 165
Colorectal surgery 162
Cone beam CT, introduction of 89
Confident 163
Congenital heart defects 148
Contaminated milk, ingestion of 94
Continuum of risk 45
Contouring radiation volumes 87
Contralateral breast cancer 167
Conventional radiation 90
Core biopsy 46, 50
Coroner's court 13
Correctness 28, 29, 31
Corticosteroids 105
Cranial nerve 57
    palsy 168
Craniofacial reconstruction 148
C-reactive protein 117
Cricoid cartilage 69
Crohn's disease 97
    during pregnancy surgery for 106
    management after intestinal resection 164
    medication used for symptom control in 106
    obstetric factors in pregnant women with 107
    surgery for abdominal 106
    surgery for perianal 106
    surgical considerations during pregnancy 103
Crohn's endoscopic recurrence, postoperative 164
Crohn's fistulae 106
Cyclosporin 105
Cytokeratin 5 56
Cytology 38
Cytomegalovirus 97

D

Deep mycosis 97
Deliberate practice 28
Destructive injuries 74
    grade 4 and 5 78
Diabetes, type 2 162
Diaphragmatic pedicle 73

Diastolic, learning concept of 30
Diffusion-weighted imaging 118
Digital imaging and communications in medicine 144
Direct-write bioprinting utilizes 145
Disease-free survival 167
Disseminated disease 55
Double-blind confident 163
Draining gastrostomy 77
Drug-coated angioplasty balloons 169
Ductal carcinoma in situ 37
Duodenal injuries 71, 76
Duodenal injuries, high grades of 77
Duodenal injury 77
Duodenal repair during surgery 77
Duodenum 69, 71, 76, 94
    approach to 76
    drainage of closed loop of 77

E

Ear and nose reconstruction, cartilage scaffolds for 148
E-cadherin gene 46
Economy of movement 29
Edematous mucosal folds 97
Elective dissection 58
Elective invasive procedure 157
Elective neck dissection 58
Electroconvulsive therapy 18
Electrosurgical plume of diathermy 41
Emergency
    appendectomy 160
    surgery 160
        evaluation of patient-controlled analgesia 160
        routine analgesia in emergency department patients 160
Endoscopy 72
Endovascular strategy 168
Endovascular surgery 168
Entrustable professional activities 29
Epidermal growth factor receptor 91
Epigenetic mechanism 49
Episiotomy, role of 107
Ergonomics of movement 29
Ericsson's view 29
Erythrocyte sedimentation rate 117
ESMO guidance 86
Esophageal
    repair 73
    stenosis 73
    stenting for iatrogenic perforation 74
    stents use of 74
Esophagus 69, 94
    proximal part of 73
    trauma 72
    travels 70

Established techniques for intraoperative assessment 38
Ethambutol 98
External beam radiotherapy 90
Extracapsular spread 58
Extracellular matrix 146
Extrapulmonary tuberculosis 94

F

Face 69
Family practitioner 104
Faxitron MX20 40
Fecal incontinence
    number of episodes 163
    risk of 107
Fecal peritonitis 162
Fecundity and fertility 103
Femoropopliteal artery disease 169
    paclitaxel-coated balloons for 169
Fibrin 146
Fine-needle aspiration cytology 59
Fistula-associated pelvic abscesses diagnosis of 97
Fistula-in-ano 95
Fitness to practice 21
Fitts and Posner's three-stage theory
    associative, stage second 27
    autonomous, stage third 27
    cognitive, stage first 27
Folic acid metabolism 106
Food and drug administration 149
Forced deposition modeling 145
Fournier's gangrene 3
Frozen section 38, 39
Fused deposition modeling 145

G

Gallbladder patch 77
Gallstone pancreatitis 161
Gas-forming PLA, presence of 114
Gas-forming pyogenic liver abscess, incidence of 117
Gastric injuries 74
    investigations 74
    radiological investigations 74
    surgical treatment 74
Gastric wounds 75
Gastroesophageal junction, posterior 75
Gastroesophageal reflux 73
Gastrografin 71
Gastrointestinal
    TB 94
    toxicity 86
Gastrointestinal tract, upper 69
Gastrojejunostomy 77
Gelatin 146

General Medical Council 13
    implications of a complaint to 20
    referral to 20, 22
General practitioner 13, 104
General surgery
    perioperative bridging anticoagulation 157
    surgical teams 157
Genitalia 90
Genitourinary tract 94
Germline mutations 46
Gillick versus West Norfolk and Wisbech area Health authority, 1986 19
Graham omental patch 77
Gram-positive cocci 5
Granulomas 97
Gross tumor volumes on CT scan 88

H

Hamman sign 71
Haptic feedback 28
HbA1C 162
Head and neck malignancies 61
Heat dissipation 41
Hematological suppression 86
Hemorrhoidal nodules 95
Hepatobiliary surgery 111
Hepatocellular carcinoma 114
Hepato-pancreato-biliary 78
Herceptin receptor 167
Herpes simplex lesions 97
High-grade ductal carcinoma in situ 47
HPV-infected anal cancer cells 92
Human immunodeficiency virus infection 85
Human papillomavirus infection 85
Hyaluronic acid 146
Hydrogels 146
Hyperbilirubinemia 114
Hyperosmolar water-soluble contrast 71

I

Ileocecal
    region 94
    spread 97
Ileus 159
Illness behaviour questionnaire 90
Immune stimulus 92
Immunosuppressive tumor microenvironment 92
Implants 148
    bioprinting 148
    synthetic implants 148
In situ lesions 49
In situ lobular neoplasia 45
Incisional hernias 158
Infection
    chronic 73
    sites of 7

Inferior vena cava 77
Inflammatory bowel disease 103
    questionnaire 90
Infraclavicular 127
Inguinal regions 90
Ink jet technology 145
Intelligent knife 41
Intensity-modulated radiation therapy 88
Intensive care unit 78
Intercostal tissue 73
Internal jugular vein 57
International Organization of Standards 149
Interstitial brachytherapy 167
Intestinal tract 69
Intimal vessel damage 134
Intra-abdominal esophagus 73
Intraluminal T-tube 77
Invasive cancer 47
    contralateral 46
    ipsilateral 46
    of ductal 49
Invasive disease, precursor of 49
Invasive lobular carcinoma 46
Invasive malignancy, risk of developing 47
Isoniazid 98

J

Jejunostomy 78
    in high-risk repairs 73
Jejunum 94
Jugular node dissection 58
Junctional peptic ulceration 78

K

Klebsiella pneumoniae 114, 116, 119

L

Lacerations
    grade 1, serosal tear 77
    grade 2, intraluminal penetration 77
    grade 3 and 4, major lacerations 77
Laparoscopic
    and thoracoscopy 72
    cholecystectomy 32
    drainage 119
    lavage 162
    peritoneal lavage 162
    resection for rectal cancer 165
    surgery for rectal cancer 164, 165
Laparotomy 76
Large-bore sampling 50
Leonard Gillespie, a British naval surgeon 3
Leukocytosis 159
Light emitting diode 96

Index

Lightness of touch 29
Litigation 13
Liver cirrhosis 114
Lobular carcinoma in situ 45
   accepted wisdom 48
   debunking 45
   diagnosed in 45
   diagnosed on core biopsy 50
   hematoxylin and eosin-stained 46f
   high-power hematoxylin 47f
   increases the risk of malignancy 49
   multifocal and bilateral 45
   requires complete excision 50
Lobular neoplasia 45
Locoregional lymphatic drainage 55
Locoregional recurrence 167
Long-thoracic nerve 130
Loperamide 106
Loss of sensation 129
Lowenstein–Jensen culture method 96
Low-molecular-weight heparin 158
Lupus vulgaris 95
Lymph node 94
   disease 61
   dissection of 58
   metastasis 55
Lymphatic drainage of the head and neck 56
Lymphogranuloma venereum 97

M

Malignancy, detection of 41
Mammary cancer, rare form of 45
Mammographic screening in women 46
Mantoux test 96
Marginprobe 40
Martial arts 31
Medical and Dental Defense Union of Scotland 13
Medical Defense Organizations 13
Medical Defense Union 13
Medical indemnity 13
Medical litigation 15, 22
   common reasons for 14
   important legal landmarks 18
   key aspects in defending 17
Medical management
   during pregnancy 104
   preconception 104
Medical Protection Society 13
Medication
   during pregnancy 105
   in Crohn's disease for disease control 105t
Medicolegal claims 14
Memorial Sloan-Kettering 46
Meninges 94
Mental rehearsal 32
Metastasis, evidence of 55

Metastatic anal cancer trials 92
Methicillin-resistant Staphylococcus aureus 5
Methotrexate 105
Methylation 49
Metoclopramide 106
Metronidazole 106
Miliary tuberculosis 94
Mitomycin 86, 91
Modified radical neck dissection 57
Modulated using multileaf collimators 88
Molecular tests 97
Monomer, type of
   acrylate 145
   N-vinylpyrolidone 145
   styrene 145
Monomicrobial 116
Montgomery versus Lanarkshire Health Board, 2015 19
Mouth 69
Mucosal ulceration 97
Multidisciplinary structure 103
Multinational medical devices industry 143
Multiple detector computed tomography 71
Muscular atrophy 129
Mutational loss 49
Mycobacterium tuberculosis 94
   bacilli 95
   culture for 96
   direct test 98
Myocardium
   contraction of 30
   relaxation of 30
Myositis 3

N

National Audit of Anal Cancer Radiotherapy 90
National Comprehensive Cancer Network
   guidelines 61, 86
   panel 62
Neck 69, 72
   dissection 56, 61
      anterolateral 58
      central compartment 58
      for evaluation of 55
      in head and neck cancers 55
      pathological evaluation of 56
      posterolateral 58
   nodes in primary squamous cell carcinomas, management of 59fc
   positioning of 72
   surgical approach 69
Necrotizing fasciitis 3
   clinical features 6
   development of 4t
   epidemiology 4
   imaging 7

important feature of 7
investigations 7
microbiology 5
of buttocks 9f
pathophysiology 4
prognosis 11
risk factors 4
risk of 8t
treatment 9
Necrotizing soft tissue infection 3, 5
classification of 5
Neoadjuvant 86
chemotherapy 165, 167
Neointimal hyperplasia 169
Neurologic thoracic outlet syndrome 127, 129f
clinical presentation 127
conservative management 128
diagnosis 128
differential diagnosis 128
surgical management 130
Nodal metastases, presence of 55
Nonsteroidal anti-inflammatory drugs 106
Nontechnical skills in surgery 28
Nontraumatic abdominal pain, emergency surgery 160
Novel
outpatient therapy for fecal incontinence 163
techniques
for margin assessment 40
intensity-modulated radiation therapy 88
principle of 40
radiotherapy for the treatment of anal cancer 85
volume-modulated arc therapy 88
Nucleic acid amplification assays 98

O

Objective structured assessment of technical skills 32
Oligomers 145
Ondansetron 106
Open repair strategy for ruptured abdominal aortic aneurysms 168
Open surgery for rectal cancer 164
Operative planning 147
Optical imaging 41
Oral cavity 55
primary tumor of 60
Organ
operating on 28
transplantation 85
Orogastric tube 72
Oropharynx, primary tumors of lateral part 60

P

Paclitaxel 92
Palpation-guided surgery 39

Pancreas 97
Pancreaticoduodenal structures, massive disruption of 76
Panitumumab 91
Paracetamol 106
Patient information 147
Patient-controlled analgesia, use of 160
Pectoralis major spasms 128
Pelvic inflammation 103
Pelvic lymph nodes 86
Penetrating trauma of upper gastrointestinal tract 69
diagnosis of injury 70
incisions and procedures 72
investigations 71
practical notes on surgical management 69
repair techniques 73
Percutaneous
drainage 118
tibial nerve stimulation 163
transluminal angioplasty 169
Perianal
cutaneous tubercular lesions 95
disease, active 103
lesions suspicious of tuberculosis, diagnosis of 99
sepsis management of 106
TB diagnosis of 97
tissues 86
tuberculosis
classification of 96t
clinical features of 95
manifestations of 94
pathogenesis of 95
Peritoneum 94
Perivascular invasion 58
PET-CT 56
Pharynx 55, 69
Pilonidal sinus 95
Planning target volume 88
Pleomorphic lobular carcinoma in situ 48f
Pleura 94
Pleural cavity, left 73
Pneumothorax 70
Polyjet printing 145
Polymerase chain reaction 97, 99
Polymicrobial 5, 116
Portable ultrasound 39
Postoperative nausea and vomiting, prevention or treatment of 158
Poststenotic dilatation distal 136
Primary tumor, treatment of 55
Programmed cell death-1 92
Prostheses 148
Prosthetic devices 148
Proton beam therapy 90
Proton-pump inhibitors 106
Pseudopolyps 97

Pulmonary TB 98
    respiratory secretions in 98
Punctate patterns 48
Pyloric exclusion 77
Pyogenic liver abscess 113
    arising from foreign body 115f
    bacteriology 116
    case series reporting on 113
    classification of 114
    diagnosis 117
    drainage tube study cholangiogram 116f
    etiology 114
    gas-forming 117f
    in patient following
        endobiliary stenting 115f
        multiple transarterial chemoembolization 115f
    investigations 117
    management 136
    principles of treatment 118
    prognosis 119
    risk factors 114
    surgery 119
Pyrazinamide 98

R

Radiation 85
Radiation Therapy Oncology Group 90
Radiation toxicity 86
    acute 87f
Radical neck dissection 57
Radiofrequency ablation 113
Radiological, histological correlation 50
Radiometric Bactec 460 TB system 96
Radiotherapy
    delivery methods, advanced 88
    techniques, developments in 88
Randomized controlled trials, recent review of 157
Rapid evaporative ionization mass spectrometry 41
Rapid immunochromatographic assay 98
Reaffirmed 5-FU 91
Rectal
    cancer 164
    stricture 95
    submucosal tumor 95
Rectum 94
Recurrent perianal lesions 95
Regulations 149
Renal failure 114
Residual disease, detection of 56
Retromolar trigone 61
Retroperitoneum 69
Rifampin 98
Right subclavian artery 135f
Robotic surgery 165
Rotator cuff injuries 128

Routine cavity shave margins 39
Routine cavity shaves 38
Roux-en-Y duodenojejunostomy 78
Roux-en-Y gastric bypass 162
Royal College of Obstetrics and Gynaecology 104
Royal College of Surgeons of Ireland 28
Royal Colleges of Surgeons 31
Ruptured abdominal aortic aneurysm 168

S

Sarcoidosis 97
Scalene 128
Scar tissue 130
Selective laser sintering 145
Sentinel lymph node sampling role of 61
Serum alkaline phosphatase 117
Sham electrical stimulation for the treatment of fecal incontinence 163
Shotgun pellets 75
Shoulder disability 61
Shoulder function impairment 60
Shoulder syndrome 57
Sigmoid colon 94
Sigmoidectomy, perforated diverticulitis 162
Simulation
    exercises 28
    models 28
    techniques 27
Skills, acquisition model of 29
Skin
    telangiectasia, late effects of 87f
    toxicity 90
    vesicles 6
Skip metastasis 60
Sloane project analysis of LN 51
Sloane project series 48
Soft tissue
    density, masses of 97
    infection 4
Spinal accessory nerve 57
Spleen 97
Squamous anal tumor 86f
Squamous cell anal cancer 91
Squamous cell carcinoma, cases of 55
Staphylococcus aureus 5
Stereolithography 145
Sterility assurance level 150
Sternocleidomastoid muscle 57
Sternomastoid muscle 69, 73
Stomach 69, 94
Streptococcus pyogenes 5
Stroma 49
Study to Optimize Peritoneal Infection Therapy trial 159
Subclavian artery 125, 134

Subclavian vein 125
    anterior aspect of 132*f*
Subclavius muscle 125, 126
Subcutaneous tissue 6
Submandibular salivary gland 57
Sulfonamides 106
Super selective neck dissection, level IIB dissection and role of 60
Superselective neck dissection 61
Supraomohyoid neck dissection 57, 60
Surgery for early stage cancers 62
Surgical
    decompression of thoracic outlet 127
    excision with upgrade 50
    skills, acquisition of 27
    teaching and training 147
    technical skills, acquisition of 33
    training
        cornerstone of 32
        environment 27
Surveillance, epidemiology and end results database 45
Symptomatic carotid stenosis 168
Syphilis 97

T

Tacrolimus 105
Tamoxifen 167
Technical skills
    assessment of 32
    attainment of 29
Technical surgical skill 29
Tension and stricture free repair 77
Terminal duct lobular unit 45
Tetracyclines 106
Thal patch 77
Thalidomide 105
Thiopurines 105
Thoracic esophageal injuries 70
Thoracic esophagus 70, 73
Thoracic outlet syndrome, anatomy of 125
    cervical ribs 126
    first rib 126
Three-dimensional Cartesian coordinate system 144
Three-dimensional printing
    in surgery, use of 143
    methodology 143
        bioinks and bioprinting 146
        direct-write bioprinting 146
        image capture and processing 144
        printing extrusion 145
        printing light polymerization 145
        printing powder bed 145
Thromboembolism, high-risk of 158
Thrombus formation 134
Tissue biopsy, histopathology of 97
Tissue loss 73, 75

Tongue
    cancers 61
    dissection 60
    primary lesions of 60
Trachea 69
Tracheobronchial
    anomalies 148
    injury 71
Tracheoesophageal fistula 73
Transarterial chemoembolization 113
Transplanted kidney 85
Traumatic tracheoesophageal fistulas, cases of 74
Treitz, ligament of 69, 76, 77
Tribunal hearings 22
Tubercle bacilli 94
Tuberculin skin test 96
Tuberculosis 99
Tumor
    cells 40, 166
    emboli in lymphatics 58
    necrosis factor 105
    specimen 41

U

UK flexible sigmoidoscopy screening trial 165
Ulcerative neoplasms 97
Upper gastrointestinal surgery 161

V

Vaginal tears risk of 107
Vaizey incontinence scores 90
Vascular
    anastomosis 32
    injury 114
    surgery 168
Venous thoracic outlet syndrome 131
    clinical presentation and diagnosis 131
    management 131
Venous thromboembolism 158
Volume modulated arc therapy 89*f*

W

Warfarin therapy 157
Weakness 129
Whipple pancreaticoduodenectomy, operating theater for 78
Whipple's procedure 116
Wounds in plastic surgery, treatment of 148

X

Xpert MTB/RIF assay 98

Z

Ziehl–Neelsen 96